Pets in Prospect

Pets in Prospect

Malcolm D. Welshman

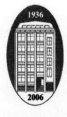

ROBERT HALE · LONDON

Typeset in 10/12½pt Janson
Printed and bound in Great Britain by
Biddles Limited, King's Lynn

Dedicated with love to my wife, Maxeen, daughter
Rebecca, and grandson, Rufus.

Chapter 1

I had been whistling a tune from *The Sound of Music* when I left Prospect House last week: *Odl lay ee. Odl lay hee hee.*

How foolish. How naïve of me. What a silly little goatherd.

Now here I was, the following Monday morning, with the waiting-room, not the hills, alive with the sound of ... dogs snuffling and whining, cats miaowing and yowling and several budgerigars chirruping and screeching. Hardly Julie Andrews with her Von Trapp family. But then I was hardly Julie Andrews even though I had a gold stud in each earlobe, hair – brown not fair – down to my collar, and a voice which would rise an octave or two when provoked.

No. I was a vet. A new graduate. And this was my first day in practice. To think I was about to unleash myself on someone's unsuspecting pet. Quite sickening really – well, for the pet anyway. If he wasn't already ill he soon would be if he knew this novice vet was about to prod and poke him. 'Now my lad, get a grip,' I said to myself. 'You've spent five years getting qualified for this moment. Now go for it. Show them what you're made of.'

So I got a grip. Only the door knob in my hand at that precise moment failed to turn as my palm was too sweaty. I gripped harder, turned it and pushed at the waiting-room door; it gave way and I tumbled into the room like a startled stoat. There was an immediate hush.

An aged spaniel gave me a rheumy-eyed stare. A chihuahua disgorged a lump of yellow froth onto its owner's shoe. Two cats bared their teeth in silent hisses. Then the chihuahua, his throat unblocked, broke the silence with a barrage of staccato yaps. Taking this as his cue to join in, the elderly spaniel lifted his head and started howling at the fluorescent light above him; he was accompanied by a chorus of cats whose plaintive wails rolled round the room like a Mexican wave.

My feeble 'Mr Kingston?' was drowned on its first syllable.

I tried again, louder, flapping my hand as if trying to summon a taxi, not someone's pet. 'Mr Kingston?'

The spaniel stopped in mid howl, wagged his tail and pulled eagerly forward on his lead. His owner yanked him back. 'Not you, stupid,' he said.

A diminutive lady cowered in her chair, engulfed by a large wicker basket that wobbled on her knees. 'Don't worry,' she crooned through the bars. 'It's not us. We're going to see that nice lady vet, Dr Sharpe.'

A woman in the far corner poked the youth sitting next to her. 'Hey, Darren, it's us 'e wants.'

The youth continued to sit there, eyes closed, head swaying rhythmically from side to side, plugged in to an iPod clipped to the belt of his jeans. The woman pulled the plug out of one of his ears and smiled across at me. 'Coming,' she shouted.

The spaniel cocked his head, and with a grizzle of expectation lunged towards her. The owner pulled him back with another 'Not you stupid.'

The woman kicked the youth's shin and he shuffled to his feet with a scowl. Between them, they manoeuvred a large metal cage past the opaque-eyed spaniel who scrabbled forward again with an eager 'woof' only to be yanked back. Once in the consulting-room, they heaved the cage onto the table. The youth quickly plugged himself in again and stood there sashaying from one foot to the other as rap music hissed faintly from his iPod.

'Tell 'im, Darren,' said the woman, giving him another prod in his ribs. The teenager continued to nod his head and jiggle his hips.

I felt myself beginning to sway and nod in unison with him while at the same time giving him an encouraging smile. Maybe he thought I was taking the mickey because he suddenly stopped jiggling and spoke. 'It's Fred. He can't eat proper.'

I pulled myself together. 'Right. Let's take a look at Fred then. See what the problem is.' Whatever Fred was, he was going to be small fry. No big fish for me. But then perhaps I was expecting too much on my first day. Rather like last week.

My expectations when I'd turned up for the interview at Prospect House had been high. I'd felt in fine fettle. Full of the spirit of youth. Well at least as much as a 25-year-old veterinary graduate can hold, with a large overdraft burning a hole in my pocket – reflecting the knee-holed jeans I normally wore – remnants of my cool image. Much better dressed today of course. Open-necked white shirt. Linen jacket. Cream chinos. I felt a bit Noël Cowardish. A mad dog, no: an Englishman, yes. And certainly one out in the midday sun.

It was a glorious June afternoon. Everywhere, roses in full bloom, though those in the front garden of Prospect House looked rather tired. Distressed even. Straggly stems, leaves pitted with black spot, a pink scattering of isolated blooms. But nothing a good dose of manure couldn't put right.

The taxi driver from Westcott-on-Sea's station knew Prospect House well. 'Ah, yes, the veterinary hospital,' he declared. 'Had my Billy Boy's bits removed there. They provided a good service. Something he can no longer do.' There was a great bellow of laughter as he slapped the steering wheel. When he dropped me off at the gates of the hospital, he leaned out of the window. 'Good luck. But watch your step,' he warned. 'That Dr Sharpe in there, she's a formidable lady by all accounts. Wouldn't want to needle her. Get it? Needle her … Sharp, eh?' With another loud guffaw, he tooted his horn and sped off.

His warning about Dr Sharpe blunted my spirits somewhat. As I climbed the short flight of stone steps to the front door, the austere portico cast a deep shadow over me, depressing me even further. Ever the one with a highly developed imagination, I felt as if I were about to enter some Doric temple and be sacrificed at the feet of the omnipotent Dr Crystal Sharpe. A gambling tryst of nymphs and satyrs on the frieze would have restored my lighter mood. But no, not a bit of it. The Victorian Worthy who had built this house had decreed the lintel be carved with a plain inscription: 'Prospect House'. I wondered just what my prospects were likely to be as I took a deep breath and stepped inside only to collide with the stooping figure of a girl wiping the floor with a mop.

'Whoops. Sorry,' I spluttered, recovering my balance to edge round her.

She looked up with a shy smile on her freckled face, her hazel eyes full of apology. She was about to speak when a voice cut in from the reception desk.

'Can I help?' The tone was brisk and demanding.

I tiptoed gingerly across the wet vinyl. 'I've come for an interview.'

The woman behind the computer screen twisted her head to one side and fixed me with a beady eye. She had bottle-black hair which was so stiffly permed and lacquered it gleamed like a polished nugget of coal. A loosely cut black jacket over a black roll-neck sweater hung round her shoulders.

'I see,' said the woman, pecking at her lapels with long, claw-like nails. 'Well, I'm afraid Dr Sharpe has had to dash out on an emergency visit. But Mr Sharpe is around somewhere.'

'Eric's in the second consulting-room,' volunteered the girl who'd been mopping down the floor. 'Shall I go and get him?' She stood up and pushed back a wisp of blonde hair.

'OK Lucy. Tell him Mr...?'

'Mitchell ... Paul Mitchell.'

'Tell Eric Mr Mitchell's here about the job.' The receptionist waved a vermilion-painted nail at Lucy who then hurried off down the corridor. 'We're all called by our Christian names here,' she said on the assumption I required an explanation. 'Makes for a more friendly atmosphere. I'm Beryl. Beryl Wagstaff.' Again she fixed me with her right eye while the left one seemed to be focused on a spot above my head. Friendly? There was nothing friendly in the eye staring at me. Cold. Glassy. Very unnerving.

Seconds later, a short, rotund figure bounced into reception, white coat open, flapping round his ankles, both arms flexing and extending in front of him as if juggling imaginary balls. The 'Pleased to meet you' faded rapidly from his lips as he skidded on the wet vinyl and careered into the desk.

'Streuth, Beryl, this floor's lethal,' he exclaimed.

'Blame it on that last client of yours, Eric,' she replied. 'The poodle cocked his leg while Mrs Pettigrew paid her bill.'

'Typical, eh?' grinned Eric Sharpe turning to me. 'And to think she was complaining the dog hadn't peed for two days.' He extended a hand and warmly shook mine. 'You've come about the job.'

I nodded.

'Good ... good. Let's go down to the consulting-room and have a chat.'

I followed the bobbing figure down the corridor into a room equipped with a gleaming stainless-steel trolley, glass-fronted wall cabinet and spotless white-topped consulting table.

'Now then,' Eric said, drawing a stool from under the table and perching himself on it, his legs swinging freely beneath him. 'Are you any good with the knife?'

I hesitated. What could I say? I'd very little opportunity to do much surgery during my training.

But he didn't wait for a reply. 'Plenty to get stuck into here. Like a good hack myself. But it's just finding the time.'

I was puzzled. Stuck into? Hack? Hardly scientific jargon.

Eric flashed me another smile. 'Before I forget, must apologize about the wife.'

Ah, yes. Here we go. The indomitable Dr Sharpe.

'Had to go out on an emergency call to the Richardsons. Very fussy clients. Won't have anyone except Crystal. Typical horsy types. Keep a couple of ponies. Very handy though if you do take the job as there'll be bucketloads of manure to be had.'

What planet was this man on? Had he been at the ether? Eric must have seen the bewilderment etched on my face.

'Muck's good for roses,' he said, as if this explained all.

It didn't.

Eric charged on. 'Well, no doubt you saw those roses out in the front of Prospect House.'

I nodded weakly.

'Not much to write home about are they?'

I shook my head in despair. He took that as my acknowledgement of the fact.

'Once you get a few shovelloads round those, there'll be no stop-ping them.' He flashed another smile, bouncing energetically up and down on the stool.

I intervened. 'Er, I'm sorry, Mr Sharpe, but I'm here about the assistant vet's post.'

Eric jumped off the stool, his face turning crimson. 'Oh I do apol-ogize. I thought you'd come about the gardening job. Crystal's trying to persuade me to take someone on to help in the grounds. Bit of a passion of mine. Gardening. But can't always find the time.' He ran a hand across his balding head. 'You must think me a complete idiot blathering on like that about the roses.'

'No ... no ... not at all.' Indeed I felt sorry for the poor man. He did seem the friendly sort and was trying to put me at my ease.

Eric took a deep breath. 'OK Paul, let's start again. Time's a bit short as I've got more appointments coming up soon. So how about you fire questions at me as I show you round?' With that, he shot out of the door.

As I chased after him, I learnt that Prospect House had been converted into a hospital by his wife some twenty-six or so years ago. Very front line, state of the art stuff he told me. But then that had always been Crystal's style. Dynamic. Keeping abreast of the latest developments. And always expected the best of her staff. Wouldn't stand for any nonsense. And that included the vets. Eric curled an eyebrow at me.

'But then I expect you know that anyway.' He shrugged. 'I'm well aware people know of Crystal's reputation for being a stickler. After all the veterinary profession's a small world. But don't let that put you off,' he added, in a reassuring tone.

I suddenly found my teeth were gnawing at my lower lip. Ouch.

I learnt that Eric was one of the early assistants who'd been subjected to her exacting standards.

'Must have done something right,' he said, with a chuckle. 'We've been married now these past twenty-two years and we still get on like the proverbial house on fire. Though we do have the occasional flaming row.' He gave another grin. 'You know how it is.'

I didn't. But had a sneaking feeling I'd find out soon enough if I took the post on.

As a demonstration, a small conflagration occurred when Eric confronted Beryl in reception re the mix-up over the interviews. It seems the gardener was due to be seen tomorrow and not today as Eric thought. Beryl's feathers were clearly ruffled at the suggestion it may have been her fault; but I could see Eric was a master at calming the old bird down and soon had her eating out of his hand again when he turned and said to me, 'We couldn't do without Beryl you know.'

A crimson glow spread up her scrawny neck to lose itself in a heavy pan of make-up. 'Well, I do my best,' she croaked.

'Of course you do, Beryl. You're indispensable. The place couldn't run without you.' He gave her another reassuring smile. 'Now tell me, what's tomorrow looking like?'

Beryl tapped a few buttons on the keyboard, her nails clicking across them. 'The computer says....' (No. This is not *Little Britain*, Paul. No TV comedy show.) Her good eye looked at the screen while the other stared blankly at me. 'Crystal's booked solid. As usual.' The good eye wandered back up to me. 'But that's no surprise. She's so ... so popular with the clients.'

Eric cleared his throat quietly. 'And my list? What's that like?'

'Oh, you've got stacks left.'

'And ops? Any booked for me?'

There was a sharp intake of breath. 'Not tomorrow, Eric. It's Tuesday, remember? Crystal's orthopaedic morning. She's got two pinnings, a cruciate and a patella luxation to deal with. Mandy's already got the theatre set up.'

'Yes, of course. Good of you to remind me.'

Did I detect a note of sarcasm there? A bit of irony?

Whatever, Eric turned to me, his baby-face features still wreathed in smiles, his eyes twinkling. 'The wife's a dab hand with the scalpel. Cutting-edge surgery and all that.' I quickly found myself being shunted into the operating theatre. 'It's not really my forte,' he went on. 'So I'm happy to leave all the complicated stuff to her. But I don't mind doing the odd spay or castration. Just to keep my hand in.'

We were now standing in front of a very complicated-looking anaesthetic machine. As if reading my thoughts, Eric said, 'Looks a bit of a monster, doesn't it?'

I nodded and fiddled absentmindedly with one of the knobs. There was a sharp pfss and the needle on the nitrous-oxide cylinder gauge shot up.

Eric appeared not to notice. 'But don't worry. Mandy, our senior nurse, is in control of all the anaesthetics. Knows what she's doing. Got high standards. But then, of course, she was trained by Crystal. So it's what you'd expect.'

The needle on the nitrous-oxide gauge continued to register escape of gas despite my furtive efforts to turn it off. I began to feel light-headed. Funny. Very funny. What a laugh this all was.

The theatre door suddenly swung open and a head popped round. 'Everything all right?'

'Ah, Mandy,' exclaimed Eric. 'Let me introduce you to—'

'M-M-Mitchell,' I interrupted, my voice high and squeaky as I tried to fight back an attack of giggles. No use. 'P-P-P-Paul Mitchell?' I squealed, feeling my lips crease back in an idiotic grin. 'Pleased to meet you … hee … hee … hee….'

There was the sharp click of heels across the polished floor as Mandy marched over to the anaesthetic machine and snapped off the valve I had been playing with. A plump, round-faced girl, she looked a picture of prim efficiency in her starched green uniform and bob of neat, auburn hair. She arranged her generous lips into a thin smile before turning to rearrange the endotracheal tubes with which Eric had started to play nervously, placing them back into their neat rows,

graded in size. 'Anything you'd like to ask me?' she queried, giving
me a hard stare that said 'This is no laughing matter, mate'.

My light-headiness evaporated in an instant.

Eric came to my rescue. 'Thanks, Mandy. But I think we've dealt
with everything now.'

He and I tiptoed out of the room leaving Mandy minutely
checking the anaesthetic machine for signs of further tampering. I
half expected her to whip out a duster and start polishing its knobs.

Eric rolled his eyes up as the theatre door swung to behind us.
'Don't be put off. Mandy's excellent at her job. Hopefully, she and
our new recruit, Lucy Gentle, should make a good team.'

I remembered the blonde-haired girl who'd been mopping down
the reception floor and the shy smile she'd given me.

'Lucy's just joined us as a trainee nurse,' explained Eric. 'Pleasant
enough girl. Just a bit reserved. But with Mandy's help, she'll no
doubt find her feet.'

Back in the office, I had just taken a mouthful of lukewarm tea
when there was the swish of tyres in the drive; the deep growl of an
engine cut out, a door slammed; a voice vibrated through reception,
the tone pitched to shatter a decanter at forty paces. 'Have I missed
him?' There was a murmured response from Beryl.

'Sounds like Crystal's back,' said Eric.

The mug in my hand jumped as the office door swung open and
in swept Dr Crystal Sharpe BVetMed, BSc, PhD, MRCVS.

Although I had never met her, I had, of course, already formed a
mental picture of this formidable lady. Her impressive qualifications
alone made her worthy of the title of 'Doctor'. But not a Dr Dolittle.
Definitely not. I was thinking more in terms of an Agatha Christie
sleuth. A tweed-clad, brogue-shod veterinary Miss Marple, black bag
in one hand, stethoscope swinging in the other, ready to track down
and treat illness in any cat or dog that dared to cross her beastly path.

How wrong I was.

The woman who swirled to a halt in front of me in a cloud of delicate perfume was far removed from that crusty old image. I was
drawn to Crystal Sharpe immediately. In fact, if this Julie Andrews
look-alike could have taken me by the hand, whisked me out of the
office and up onto the Downs with a burst of *Climb Ev'ry Mountain*,
I'd have been a very happy goatherd.

'You must be Paul Mitchell,' she said, in a clipped mid-shire's
accent.

I found my hand clasped by hers, slim fingers, short, well-mani-cured nails, devoid of varnish. Her face too was unblemished by make-up. Laughter lines sprang from the corners of intense steel-blue eyes, eyes which at that moment were boring uncomfortably into mine. Dainty pearl studs adorned petite earlobes below fringed, short tresses of copper curls. A perfect English rose? Maybe. But wasn't there a thorny side to this lady?

The hand unclasped itself and an apology made.

'Sorry I wasn't here to meet you. But I'm sure Eric was able to give you some idea how we operate.'

I felt myself blush, remembering my giggling fit in the theatre.

Her husband's face lit up with another cheery smile. 'We covered most things,' he said, putting a finger to his lips and giving me a conspiratorial wink.

'And, of course, we've studied your CV very thoroughly,' added Dr Sharpe. 'So...?' She was again scrutinizing my face. 'Are you prepared to take the post?'

My mind was still leaping goat-like over alpine meadows. I should have been asking more questions. What happened to the last assis-tant? Why did he leave so quickly? Why were they so desperate for a replacement? But my head was up in the clouds. And mesmerized by Crystal's piercing blue eyes, I said 'Yes' without thinking.

Minutes later I found myself skipping down the drive of Prospect House whistling *Edelweiss* having promised to start the following week.

Seven days later, I'd plummeted down from those alpine slopes onto the more earthly terrain of the second consulting-room in Prospect House where I was peering into a cage stuffed with bars, swings, wheels and tunnels.

'Fred's a bit of an escape artist,' explained the woman, as her son unlocked the three padlocks on the cage door; he then stood back, reconnected himself to his iPod and started rocking on the spot again.

There was what looked like a nest box up in the far right-hand corner of the cage.

'He'll be in there,' said the woman, catching my quizzical look.

Only with my whole arm crammed in up to my shoulder, elbow wedged in the bottom corner, could I get my fingers anywhere near the nest box. I cautiously inserted three fingers. What was I going to find? I felt the prickle of straw, the warmth of fur and then suddenly the pain of a creature's teeth sinking into my index finger.

'Ouch.' My hand shot out of the nest box bringing with it a tan ball of fur which held on grimly, bouncing through the rodent playground as I extricated my arm from the cage. I inadvertently flicked my wrist. The tan ball sailed over my shoulder and crashed into the instrument trolley scattering scissors and scalpels.

I pounced. 'Got you,' I said. But missed.

Fred nimbly scuttled between the bottles of antibiotics. The youth stopped jigging to nonchalantly step round the consulting table and scoop Fred into his palm before dropping him into mine with a 'Here, mate.'

I mouthed my thanks and stared down at my first patient. Fred the hamster. Not exactly a giant of the pet kingdom. More a titch. Had five years of intense study really accumulated in me being given the beady eye by this tiny little rodent? I scruffed the creature and turned him over. His eyes bulged. His whiskers twitched. With lips parted, two long yellow incisors curled down like scimitars.

I scrabbled with my left hand for the nail clippers. Two snips and the teeth were restored to normal length.

'He'll be able to eat now,' I said. I should have added 'And nip now,' since I suddenly felt Fred test his teeth by sinking them into my finger. They were sharp, very sharp – making me feel quite needled.

Beryl's eye was quick to spot the splattering of blood on my white coat as I ushered Fred and co. out into reception, my bitten finger crossed in an attempt to staunch the blood still dripping. 'Paul,' she warned, 'I should get out of that coat before—'

'Before I catch sight of you.' The voice of Maria – sorry, Crystal – sang through the air. But it was far from melodious. By its icy tone I was clearly not one of her favourite things.

Startled, I jumped round to find Crystal standing in the doorway of the office, arms folded, every pore oozing disapproval.

'I think you'd better come in here a minute,' she went on.

Beryl cast me a pitiful look as I trailed across like some errant schoolboy approaching the headmaster's study. I sensed I was about to face the music; but not the sound of music I wanted to hear.

Chapter 2

In the event, my anticipated hauling over the coals by Crystal turned out to be no more than a gentle admonishment. She'd been anxious to make sure I replaced my blood-splattered coat before seeing my next patient.

'I realise you're just finding your feet,' she'd said.

And hamsters just finding my fingers, I thought, my bitten index finger still throbbing.

'Don't hesitate to change coats whenever you need to,' she went on. 'Mandy will always oblige.' She gave the sweetest of smiles.

Oh that smile. Then, as in the future, I found myself zooming up an Austrian mountain as those coral pink lips curved and those soft, apple cheeks dimpled. Do Re Mi. Far – a long, long way to run? Yes. But definitely worth it. Crystal could light up my life any time. My Ray … my drop of golden sun.

As for Mandy. Doe … a dear? No way. I soon found out she was the mother superior of Prospect House. No novice nun was she. No Maria.

'Another coat … so soon?' she'd queried when I'd nipped down to the laundry room to ask for a replacement. Her spotless, crisp, creaseless habit (uniform) positively crackled with displeasure. The look she gave me nearly had me on my knees, clasping the gold chain round my neck – a small one, nothing too chunky, I wasn't medallion man – while begging for forgiveness.

Beryl, on the other hand, tried to keep a motherly, less superior eye on me. Just the one eye as it happened. Eric was later to tell me that she'd lost her right eye in a childhood accident and had it replaced by an artificial one.

'And be warned,' Eric said, 'if she gets flustered, it's likely to fall out. Then everything grinds to a halt while we scrabble around looking for it. Almost got swallowed by a spaniel once. So do keep an eye on her. Preferably two.'

Beryl certainly gave me a look every time I arrived for work. I'm not sure whether she disapproved of the gold studs in my ears, the gold necklace or my highlighted hair. Maybe she just thought my chinos were a little too tight and my short-sleeved shirt a little too shocking pink. Whatever, I was eyeballed daily.

Still, she did try to ease me into the routine at Prospect House. Usually there were two consulting-rooms in use simultaneously. I was allocated the smaller, darker one overlooking the exercise yard. Eric and Crystal used the larger, sunny room overlooking the rose garden. Eric and I did morning and evening consultations, Crystal a smattering of early afternoon ones.

'Time for her special clients,' Beryl informed me. 'When she's not being requested to visit them, that is. Like Lady Derwent for instance. She's specifically asked for Crystal to make a house visit. Her Labradors need their annual boosters.' To emphasize the point, that morning, she drew a long vermilion nail across the computer screen where 'Lady Derwent – Warren Place' had been typed in capitals with CMS alongside. 'But don't look discouraged, Paul,' she went on.

Me? Look discouraged? Well, maybe I was looking a little down in the mouth. But hey, come off it, Paul, I'm the new boy. My chance will come one day. Do Re ... for Me. For when I've made a name for myself.

'You may find the next client interesting. A Miss McEwan,' said Beryl, twisting her head towards me, her heavily painted lips pulling back, their corners disappearing into her cheeks. 'She's got a—'

Further words were lost as the reception-room door swung open and in sailed a diminutive woman, like an out-of-control kite, her body encased in a tartan cape which billowed from her tiny shoulders and flapped round her booted ankles. 'Dear me,' she cried, her voice high pitched, shrill. 'It's blowing a gale out there. Who'd have thought ... late June.' She spun to a halt in the middle of reception, her neck craning from the cape like a jerking pigeon on the look-out for crumbs. Her beady eye caught Beryl's glassy one. 'I wonder if someone would be kind enough to fetch Cedric out of the car for me. He's a bit difficult to manage on my own. It's the old hands, you see.'

As if to demonstrate, her arms flew out from the folds of the red cape and, palms forward, she waved her hands at shoulder-level. Any minute I expected her to burst out into song. *My old Mammie* perhaps? There seemed to be a full set of digits on each hand so I guessed she was talking about a touch of arthritis.

I didn't wait to find out, leaving Beryl to sort out the situation while I melted back into my dingy consulting-room made more dingy by a Virginia creeper growing out-of-control round the window. Still it helped to block the view of the adjacent exercise yard which, I was to discover, always smelt foul even though constantly being doused down with disinfectant. The malodorous air constantly permeated the room and made clients sniff and eye me suspiciously as soon as they entered.

When Miss McEwan's records flashed up on the computer screen I scrolled down through her details. OK. She owned a collie called Ben. He seemed to have a long clinical history. It went on for pages. Then abruptly stopped six months ago. Put to sleep with terminal cancer. Oh dear. But then maybe this Cedric I was about to see was his replacement? A sweet new puppy requiring his vaccinations?

I jumped at the sound of metal crashing into the door.

'Do be careful, dear. You'll upset Cedric,' trilled Miss McEwan as Lucy, her face beetroot, wisps of hair floating free from her pony-tail, struggled in, arms wide apart, hands clutching the sides of a large blue metallic bird cage, covered in a red tartan blanket matching Miss McEwan's cape.

'Meet Cedric,' gasped Lucy. 'If you need any help just shout.' She gave me a shy smile and then slipped out to leave me with Miss McEwan's coal-black eyes staring out from a face with the complexion of a once used tissue. She gave a sniff and looked round as if wondering where the smell was coming from before saying, 'Cedric's very special, you know.'

I slid the blanket off the cage and found myself being stared at by another set of coal-black eyes. Only these belonged to a bird a little larger than a blackbird and with bright yellow wattles. It hopped along the perch towards me, cocked his head and fixed me with a beady look.

Miss McEwan edged along the consulting table and did the same. 'He's very special,' she repeated, turning to the bird. 'Aren't you, Cedric?'

The bird bobbed up and down and then in Miss McEwan's precise tone of voice said 'Cedric's special.'

Miss McEwan gave a high-pitched tinkle of a laugh. 'Yes, you are, pet. Let's hope this vet knows how to treat mynahs.'

I didn't actually. We briefly covered the workings of a chicken at veterinary college and I once poked a dead blackbird I'd found on my parent's lawn; hardly the stuff of avian medicine. The nearest I'd got to operating on a bird was pulling the giblets out of an oven-ready chicken. Cedric gave me a startled look and rapidly hopped away.

Miss McEwan addressed me. 'They're not like cats or dogs, you know.'

I did know. Five years of veterinary training had at least taught me that. I took a deep breath and rather pompously said, 'I am familiar with the avian species.' I could have added 'Roasted at gas mark 6 with sage and onion stuffing.' But somehow thought Miss McEwan would find the comment in poor taste. So I tried to be tactful. 'You say his name's Cedric?'

'Ask him,' shrilled Miss McEwan.

'Sorry?'

'Ask him. Go on. He wouldn't mind. It's his party piece.'

I groaned inwardly. This was all I needed. A tête-à-tête with a mynah bird. But maybe this was all part of establishing a good rapport with clients. A new learning curve for me. So I turned to his cage and cleared my throat. 'What's your name?' I said.

The bird bounced back and forth along the perch, clearly delighted at being spoken to. But he didn't reply.

'Ask him again,' urged Miss McEwan. She saw me hesitate. 'Go on. Ask him.'

I felt a tic throb in my forehead. This was getting silly. But such was Miss McEwan's insistence I felt obliged to obey. 'What's your name?'

'What's your name?' echoed Cedric, in a perfect imitation of Miss McEwan's voice, the tone so strident I almost felt compelled to answer.

'Go on, tell him,' shrieked Miss McEwan, hopping from one foot to another, her cape flapping wildly round her shoulders.

'Paul Mitchell.'

'My name's Cedric,' said the mynah with a manic cackle.

Miss McEwan also began to laugh, a bell-like peal of laughter that rolled round the room. Cedric, mimicking his bouncing owner, jumped up and down emitting a series of piercing whistles.

Suddenly, the door swung open and Eric popped his head round, grimacing at the noise. 'Everything all right, Paul?'

'Yes … yes …' I seethed, throwing the blanket back over the cage. There was a deathly silence followed by a muffled raspberry.

'Very well then. I'll let you get on with it,' said Eric, swiftly withdrawing.

'Dear me. Cedric's a card and no mistake,' sniffed Miss McEwan, snatching a tissue from the folds of her cape to dab the corners of her eyes. The scent of lavender infused the room. 'I don't know what I'd do without him.'

'So what's the problem?' I asked tersely.

Miss McEwean snapped to attention and explained. Over the last month Cedric had been pecking at his tail. Once or twice she'd found spots of blood on the floor of his cage and realized something must be irritating him. 'Of course I keep telling him to stop but all he does is mimic me.'

From under the blanket came a muffled 'Stop it'.

'See what I mean.'

I nodded. 'Best if we take a look.' As I removed the blanket again, Cedric cocked his head and gave a wolf whistle. He gave another startled whistle as I winkled him out of the cage, his head pinned between my index and third finger, my other fingers curled over his wings. Feeling down his back, I discovered a distinct lump over the base of his tail. Parting the feathers, the lesion was obvious. A large, raised, raw area. His preening gland – the gland used to oil and keep a bird's feathers well groomed. I slid Cedric back into the cage and he flapped onto his perch with an indignant squawk. I closed the door and turned to Miss McEwan.

'There's a problem with his preening gland. Either an infection or….' I hesitated not wishing to alarm her unduly. But it had to be said. 'It could be a tumour.'

Miss McEwan gripped the edge of the consulting table, her bony knuckles blanched. Her voice dropped to a soft twitter. 'Oh dear. That sounds rather serious. Can anything be done about it?'

I gave a slight shrug and tried to inject some confidence in my reply. 'The gland can be removed. But it would mean major surgery.'

Miss McEwan peered into the cage. 'Oh dear me. Dear me. My poor Cedric.'

The mynah cocked his head. 'Poor Cedric,' he replied, his tone solemn.

I explained that we had to do something otherwise Cedric would continue to peck at the gland and make the problem worse. I was in full flow, sounding confident, sounding sure of my facts when Miss McEwan interrupted me.

'Have you operated on a bird before?'

Crash. I was instantly floored. I could feel myself going bright red. Me? A new graduate. Operated on a bird? My hesitation was enough for the wily old bird in front of me.

'You haven't, have you?'

I quickly reassured her that Cedric would be in the best possible hands. Dr Crystal Sharpe's hands to be precise. She of cutting fame. An expert in all things surgical. I just prayed an Indian hill mynah's rear end came within that remit. Miss McEwan was relieved when I told her.

'Could I leave Cedric with you now then?' she went on. 'It would be much easier than taking the cage all the way home and then back again. What with these.' Her hands did their hallelujah wave again.

Oh Lord. Just what was I letting myself in for?

The rest of the morning was punctuated by a piercing monologue echoing up from the ward as Cedric repeatedly shrieked, 'What's your name? My name's Cedric.'

Mandy was very put out that I'd booked an operation for later that day without first having consulted her. 'Really, Paul. It's not an emergency. It could have waited.' She stood there, arms folded over her generous bosom. Her damson eyes flashed. She was cross. Oh dear, I had sinned – a naughty novice in her nunnery. Her lips shrank into a thin line as Cedric let rip with an unholy raspberry. Least he seemed to be on my side. 'So what time do you propose doing it?'

I opened my mouth but she butted in before I had a chance to say anything. 'I suggest two o'clock. Crystal will have finished her list by then.' She looked up from the ops book, pen poised over the page. 'OK?'

'Er ... well ... I was rather hoping Crystal might do it.'

Mandy straightened up. 'Crystal?' The name hung in the air. Holy Mary. Mother of God. What had I said?

'Yes, Crystal,' I faltered, the words a mere whisper. Her disgusted look made me feel as if she'd discovered some dirty habit of mine. I fought the urge to genuflect. Oh me of little faith in myself.

'I hardly think so,' said Mandy in a very superior (no trace of mother in it) tone of voice. She scribbled my initials in the book and marched away with brisk snap of her uniform. Did she know something I didn't? Apparently so.

When Crystal returned from her visit to Lady Derwent I broached the subject. She planted a hand firmly on my shoulder, fixed me with her steely-blue eyes and said in her precise, clipped voice, 'There's one thing you have to learn here, Paul. You follow through your own cases. I'm sure it's something you'd wish to do anyway.' The hand stayed clamped to my shoulder. 'Am I right?'

'Well, it's just that I thought....'

The hand dug in tighter.

'Yes, of course.'

The hand relaxed. 'Good. See it as a challenge.'

I saw it as a potential disaster.

Five past two I was in the operating-room, gowned up, boots on and, despite the warmth of the room, shivering. When Lucy clanged in with the cage, Mandy swept in from the prep room and stopped her from placing it on her altar (operating table). 'Not on my nice clean top, thank you very much,' she said, and, pointing to an adjacent trolley, added, 'Put it there.'

Lucy grimaced. Hello ... hello ... did I sense a little antagonism between these two?

'What's your name?' shrieked Cedric unperturbed by Mandy's dismissive manner – though Lucy seemed a trifle ruffled.

She raised her eyebrows at me and whispered, 'Good luck' before quietly slipping out.

'Now,' said Mandy briskly. 'I've sterilized all the instruments I think you'll need.' She waved at the operating trolley.

Looking lost in the centre of a vast, green drape was a small pile of instruments consisting of a tiny pair of scissors, scalpel, fine eyebrow tweezers and some forceps normally used for eye operations.

Mandy pulled the anaesthetics trolley round to the side of the table and from the labyrinth of valves, bottles and pipes, plucked out a narrow black tube which ended in a rubber cone. She snaked it onto the table and fastened it down with a sandbag, checked the level of halothane, adjusted the valve setting slightly and then declared herself ready to start.

I quickly looked round the room to make sure all the windows and doors were closed.

'I've already checked,' said Mandy.

Grrrr … I picked up a towel and turned to the cage. Opening the door, I pounced on Cedric, enfolded him in one swoop, and scooped out the wriggling bundle.

'My name's Cedric,' he spluttered, as I levered his head out of the towel and Mandy plunged the cone over his beak.

'Sleepy-byes for you, Cedric,' she said in a no-nonsense tone of voice – a tone I was to become all too familiar with over the subsequent months. She turned up the flow of the halothane-oxygen mixture with a deft twist of the valve.

I felt Cedric's chest heaving through the towel. There was a rattle of beak against cone as he shook his head, fighting against the anaesthetic. Suddenly he went still. I relaxed my grip, uncertain as to what was happening. Then in Miss McEwan's precise, tinkling voice, Cedric exclaimed, 'You're a dirty dick.'

I just collapsed with laughter. In doing so my grip on the towel slackened. It was enough. Cedric wriggled free and with ruffled black feathers sticking out in all directions, hopped across the operating table, paused, then sprung onto the instruments where he promptly lifted his tail and relieved himself.

Mandy was far from amused. Didn't see the funny side of it at all. 'Oh really, Paul,' she snapped , turning off the anaesthetics machine while I tried to wipe the smile off my face.

With a quavery wolf-whistle, Cedric lurched off the trolley and skidded onto the floor where he waddled like a pickled duck towards the prep room. Fighting back another wave of giggles, I ran round the ops table, towel in hand, and pinned him down. But not before he'd left a liquid trail behind him.

'What a mess,' declared Mandy, her face like a slab of unleavened dough, not a crack of a smile evident.

A muffled raspberry made me start quaking again. I squeezed my lips together desperate not to let a snort of laughter escape as under Mandy's steely gaze, I popped Cedric back in his cage. I was only allowed to start the operation again once everything had been mopped down, disinfected and the instruments resterilized.

'OK, matey,' I declared. 'Second time lucky.' With Cedric's head this time safely secured in the cone, he slipped into unconsciousness with a series of sleepy wolf-whistles.

Mandy then whisked the towel away, stretched him out, taped down his wings and deftly plucked the feathers from around the preening gland. I was actually grateful for her obvious expertise. At least someone knew what they were doing. When she'd finished, she stepped back. 'You can start now,' she instructed.

Yes, ma'am, here goes then, I thought, my fingers hovering over the tiny pile of instruments. The ugly mass of red tissue took some cutting out. Blood welled up from the wound and soaked into the drapes.

Mandy leaned over and sniffed. 'It's bleeding rather a lot.'

I was only too aware of the fact. The haemorrhage did seem rather excessive. If nothing else, I did know birds couldn't afford to lose too much of their blood volume and here was Cedric's vital fluids draining into the drapes. Would he survive me poking around like this? Would he survive the shock? I pressed on, beads of sweat coursing down my arms as the circle of blood grew wider.

'You may find this of help.' Mandy held up a bottle. 'It's dissolvable gauze. Crystal finds it useful. Not that she gets much bleeding.'

Grrrr....

She tipped some out onto the operating trolley.

By now I'd dissected out the preening gland – or at least the blob of tissue that vaguely resembled it. What was left was a ragged hole which rapidly filled with blood every time I swabbed it out. I was grateful for the gauze; and rammed a wodge of it into the crimson crater, pressing it firmly in, before stitching a flap of skin across.

With Cedric returned to his cage to lie on a pad of cotton-wool, Mandy summoned Lucy to take him back to the ward while she, as she put it, 'cleaned up the mess'. It was said with just the merest flicker of her long eyelashes in my direction.

I helped Lucy manoeuvre the cage onto a table next to a radiator in the ward and then stood back, biting my lower lip, looking at the limp bird stretched out on the pad, waiting for him to come round from the anaesthetic.

'He'll be OK,' said Lucy, trying to sound reassuring. 'You'll see.'

And I did see. Within ten minutes, Cedric had started to twist and turn, his wings flapping, his legs waving in the air. Within a further five, he was wobbling about his cage, trying to climb up the bars and falling off at every attempt. After twenty minutes he had made it to his perch and sat there swaying. He looked at us bleary-eyed and in a croaky voice uttered his first post-operative 'What's your name?'

Lucy's freckled face lit up. 'There. What did I tell you?'

I still wasn't convinced. OK, Cedric had got through the operation. But the next twenty-four hours would be crucial to his survival.

*

I phoned through to the hospital that evening. Lucy was on duty.

'Cedric's fine,' she informed me. 'He's not pecked at his stitches. And there's been no bleeding.'

As I put the phone down, a voice rang out from down the hallway. 'Everything all right?' It was Mrs Paget, my landlady as of last weekend, standing in the doorway of her lounge. The digs were a temporary measure until such time as the practice cottage promised me by the Sharpes became available. It was on Beryl Wagstaff's recommendation that I took the room at Mrs Paget's. She assured me I'd get a warm welcome as her friend, Cynthia, a middle-aged divorcee, apparently 'simply adored animals' and would be 'thrilled to the core to have a young vet under her roof'. I wasn't so thrilled when her chihuahua charged down the hall and gave me a savage nip on my ankle before I'd even stepped across the threshold. But being just a few hundred yards down the road from Prospect House, the lodgings were convenient; even if the pooch was a pain, as the many subsequent bites on my ankles proved.

This evening was no exception. Chico had barged up to the telephone table and was now baring his teeth waiting to pounce on any flesh I chose to expose. But I had got wise to him now and never ventured out of my room unless wearing thick socks and trainers.

It was a shame that I had to run the gauntlet of Chico's teeth in order to use the phone in the hall, but since my mobile had no signal in the house and the roar of traffic outside made conversation impossible, I found myself with no choice. I had to grit my teeth while Chico bared his.

'Just checking on one of my patients,' I explained, as Mrs Paget shuffled down the hall, cigarette dangling from the side of her mouth, and with an ineffectual wave said 'Shoo ... shoo' to an unresponsive Chico whose sole focus was on what was only two feet away. My two feet.

I retreated to my room to spend a restless night fretting about Cedric.

But all seemed well the next morning. He'd continued to leave the stitches alone and the wound was clean and dry. Miss McEwan was delighted when told she could take Cedric home.

'I can't thank you enough,' she gushed, as Lucy and I levered

Cedric's cage into the back of her Mini. 'Dr Sharpe's done such a marvellous job. Please pass on my thanks.'

Lucy's eyes widened with astonishment. 'But—'

'I certainly will,' I interjected, quickly pulling the blanket over Cedric and closing the car door. I turned to Lucy and shook my head.

Miss McEwan squeezed herself in behind the steering wheel, her head just coming level with it, her tartan cape spilling over the edges of the seat. She wound the window down. 'Now you did say to come back in a week's time?'

'A week ... yes. Unless Cedric starts pecking at the wound.'

'Most grateful. Most grateful,' she murmured, switching the engine on.

I leaned down, placing my hand on the window-sill. 'Before you go, there's one question I'm dying to ask, if you don't mind.'

Miss McEwan looked up at me. 'Well?'

'I was just wondering whether you knew anyone called Dick?'

Two high spots of red instantly appeared on Miss McEwan's cheeks and her lips rapidly drew into a moue. She revved the car and crashed into gear. I leapt back as the car lurched forward, gravel spitting from under the tyres. As it squealed out of the drive and disappeared, loud wolf-whistles rang out from the back seat.

I gave Lucy a wink as we ran giggling up the steps and into reception. We were instantly sobered by Beryl giving us the eye. Just the one – her good one.

Chapter 3

It was a morning towards the end of my second week, that Beryl asked the question. I'd been scanning my diary, checking for any visits she might have booked in.

'Are you superstitious?' she enquired.

I thought for a moment. No. I didn't really think so. I'd skirt round a ladder, but only if someone was up it with a pot of paint. But that was just common sense. And the sight of three magpies – or was it four? – I didn't see as an omen of doom. Merely successful breeding on the part of the magpies.

'Why do you ask?'

'Oh, just wondered.' Beryl rubbed a wart on her chin. 'It's just that I've booked you a visit later this morning. It's a black cat. Just thought … maybe … you know … seeing it could bring you some luck.'

I was instantly suspicious. Luck? Did I need luck? Did she know something I didn't? I knew she was friendly with Mrs Paget. Perhaps the two of them had been having a chin-wag. Comparing notes. Sizing me up. Maybe Mrs Paget had told her of my run-ins with Chico and all those disturbed nights on duty.

'I can sympathize with the poor lad,' I can hear her say. 'Keeps me awake just thinking about him.'

Yes, well, Mrs Paget. Keep those thoughts to yourself.

Mind you, she had a point. I did have a lot of night duties – a whole string of them. I'd barely stepped over the threshold of Prospect House when the roster was sorted out with what seemed like unseemly haste. I had assumed it would be shared between the three vets – like one in three. Not a bit of it. It transpired that Crystal and Eric expected me to do alternate nights. I explained this to Mrs Paget whose mascara-laden lashes whipped up and down in a frenzy when I said her nights might be disrupted.

'I don't mind a bit,' she said, stubbing out her cigarette and drawing the lapels of her housecoat across her bosom. 'It's all for a good cause. Saving our little furry friends. In fact I wish there was more I could do to help.'

She was to mull over this for a few days as I later found out.

There had been ground rules when I first began lodging with her. My bedsit was the converted lounge at the front of the house. I could use the kitchen from one to two at lunchtimes, five to seven in the evenings, including weekends. Mornings were just half-an-hour from seven-thirty.

'Otherwise you might bump into me in a state of undress,' she said.

I was unclear as to who would be the one undressed, but fearing it could be her – naked but for her fluffy pink housecoat – I stuck to the rules rigidly.

Even so getting back in time to use the kitchen in the evenings proved impossible. People came home from work to find a sick pet and would phone through asking to be seen. So consultations often ran past the allotted close of six o clock. I'd stagger back to Mrs Paget's kitchen with barely time to throw a chilli-con-carne-for-one in the microwave.

It clearly concerned Mrs Paget.

'My dear, I've been giving this some thought,' she declared, wandering into the kitchen, ashtray in one hand, cigarette in the other, to stand watching me bolt down that evening's ready meal – a fisherman's pie through which I was trawling to find a flake or two of fish. 'I can't bear the thought of you having to rush back every evening. It must be so stressful for you. I'd like to help out.'

Help? That sounded promising. A little home cooking maybe? A nice shepherd's pie with fresh vegetables from the garden waiting for me when I returned after a long and exhausting surgery?

'Yes,' she continued, dragging on her cigarette and exhaling sharply. 'I've decided to extend your permitted time in the kitchen to seven-thirty.'

Oh wow. Lady Luck (Mrs Paget) has smiled (leered wantonly) on me. Perhaps when Beryl had talked about luck she'd sensed I needed more than being offered an extra half-hour in a divorcee's kitchen to give me a boost.

*

But her idea of getting lucky by having a black cat cross my path was way off course. But then she didn't know the path I found myself treading later that morning was going to be such an overgrown one, looping through a tangle of brambles, waist-high with nettles.

'Have you spotted him yet?' trumpeted Major Fitzherbert from the safety of a much easier path – the paved one bordering his garden.

'No. Not yet,' I called back, swearing under my breath as a briar scratched a neat line of blood across the back of my right hand while another snagged my right sock. This can't be happening, surely? I thought. Me, a professional person, floundering through a sea of thorns? Certainly, Crystal or Eric wouldn't have allowed themselves to get into such a situation.

'He's in there somewhere, the little bounder,' boomed the major, his stick pounding defiantly on the paving stones.

I continued to edge my way further into the thicket, my back bending more and more with each step I took.

'Keep going, there's a good chap. Flush him out,' ordered the major.

I stooped lower, pushed forward a few more inches, arms clawing the brambles apart. This was getting ridiculous. Any minute now I'd be on my hands and knees pleading 'Puss … Puss....' Which was nonsense when I understood from Major Fitzherbert that the cat in question was a rather large black tom indisposed to human companionship.

'You mean "wild",' I'd said when the major first informed me.

'In the true sense of the word,' he stated, his voice ringing with pride. 'Fine fellow. Independent sort. Won't let anyone near him.'

Then why in hell's name was I attempting to lure the cat out of the wilderness of gorse and brambles that bordered Major Fitzherbert's garden? But that, it seemed, was the major for you. From the moment I met him, I felt compelled to obey his command. He was tall, solid, and apart from the white hair that swept back from a high, furrowed forehead, sixty-five years of living had done little to crumple the firm set of the jaw, the deep authoritative voice and the hooded, almost translucent, light-blue eyes. It was those eyes, with their penetrating unblinking stare, that dared me to defy his order to drop my black bag and scurry into the thicket like a rabbit bolting down a burrow.

'I think I saw him then,' the major barked again. 'Over to your left a bit.'

I shuffled round only to be confronted by an impenetrable barrier of gorse, a blanket of yellow blooms producing a warm pungent smell reminiscent of coconuts . 'No way through,' I yelled back.

'Nonsense!'

Over the riot of brambles, I could see the major's stick waving backwards and forwards. 'Go on man. Push through. Push.'

The major might have been used to commanding a battalion of men to make the final push through the jungles of Africa, but I was just a novice vet in the leafy suburbs of West Sussex and nothing would induce me to go further. I retreated, preferring to confront the barbs of Major Fitzherbert's tongue to the multiple lashings I was getting from the gorse and brambles. I felt the parting rasp of a brier as I struggled back to the relative safety of the border; I could feel the major's eyes on me as I carefully edged through his delphiniums and lupins – lined up like soldiers on parade. Woe betide me if I broke their ranks.

'Got away from you, did he?' crowed the major as I hopped back onto the path, plants intact, self-confidence crushed. 'He's a cunning beast. Devil of a job to outsmart him.' He thrust a hand deep into the pocket of his cavalry twill jacket, tapped his stick against his cords and then began to briskly hobble towards his cottage.

I snatched up my black bag and trotted behind him.

Halfway up the path he stopped and looked over his shoulder. 'You know what I would do, laddie?' The hooded eyes bored into me, mere slits, shadowed against the sun. 'I'd dart him. You know. Like the zoo chappie.'

I glanced down and minutely inspected the pinpricks of blood that the back of my right hand sported. Who did he think I was? Some sort of big game hunter on safari in a white topee, stalking the slopes of the South Downs for his wretched feral cat – a cat that was apparently wounded and in need of stitching? My patience, like the blood oozing from my scratches was running thin. I took a deep breath. 'A better idea would be to trap him.'

Major Fitzherbert's eyebrows knotted together like two white caterpillars head-butting. 'Trap?' The word reverberated round the garden causing several blackbirds to shoot out of the undergrowth squawking with alarm. 'Don't hold with that sort of nonsense.'

'I mean ... er ... corner him somewhere,' I faltered, feeling myself to be the one already trapped, impaled on stakes in the bottom of a pit. 'Like in a garden shed ... or....' I desperately looked round, trying to break from the hooded blue eyes that were still fixed on me. I pointed to the left of the cottage. 'Perhaps in your greenhouse over there.'

The major finally glanced away. He drew himself up to his full height, took his hand out of his jacket pocket and pulled the flap down smartly. 'Well....' he harrumphed. 'That could be one plan of action I suppose. Leo does take the occasional catnap in there.'

'Leo?'

'That's what I said, laddie. Leo. He's more of a lion than your average cat. I've always admired animals with a bit of spunk. None of this pussy-footing around with lap dogs and the like.' He gave me another hard stare before turning to march stiffly on up the path. 'Let's go and take a look, shall we? Give it the once over.'

The greenhouse was a magnificent structure, very Victorian with whorls of glass and white cast-iron tracery; its shape was reminiscent of the Albert Hall, having a central domed roof dwarfing, and quite out-of-character with, the thatch of the cottage. Nevertheless I felt compelled to make some favourable comment especially with the major breathing down my neck. I wasn't going to shirk my duty.

'What a superb greenhouse. And that central dome ... very ... er ... imposing.'

'Pleased you should say that. Most people think it's out-of-keeping. But then there are so many fuddy-duddies around here. Far too conventional the lot of them.' He gazed at the greenhouse and sighed. 'Had it built when I returned from Africa.'

To judge from the riot of palms and vines I could detect through the misty panes, he must have returned with a slice of Africa as well. The whole building was bursting at the seams with greenery. As the major slid back the door, several long, sappy tendrils flopped down over the entrance. He parted the vines and took a deep breath of the steamy atmosphere, standing motionless, for once silent. At last he snapped to and said 'Brings back the old memories. Those were the days.' He sighed. 'Does need a bit of a prune though.'

I peered into the emerald interior. Any second, I expected a humming bird to flash into view or a swallowtail flit from the dense array of white lilies, scarlet hibiscus and bowers of purple bougainvillea that ranged down each side of a central aisle, a gravelled aisle on which a basking python would not have looked out-of-place.

I stepped back. 'So you think we could trap him in there?'

The major gave another loud harrumph as he thrust the door closed. 'Your idea, laddie. Not mine.'

I persisted. 'Do you put food out for Leo?'

'I do indeed.'

'Then perhaps we could crush some pills in it.' I reached into my black bag and pulled out a vial of yellow tablets, extracting three to offer to the major.

He took them and rolled them round in his palm. 'What are they? Knock-out pills?'

'Tranquillizers.'

The major snorted. 'Still say it would be better to dart him.'

'Let's just give this a try,' I said, my voice as firm as I could make it. 'If nothing else it should make Leo drowsy.'

'Doubt if he'll take them. He's a cunning devil. Very sharp.'

'Whatever. Let's keep our fingers crossed.' Fingers crossed? What was I saying? Thought I wasn't superstitious. I left promising to return the next day providing Leo was then inside the greenhouse and had been given the doctored food. Touch wood, he would have eaten it. Touch wood? I was at it again.

My mood wasn't too good when I returned to Prospect House.

Beryl's choice of words was unfortunate. 'Any luck?' she asked.

'Just the opposite. A complete waste of time. Didn't even see the creature.'

Beryl lowered her good eye and discretely rebooked the visit for the following day. Major Fitzherbert phoned that afternoon to insist I made it 11.30 on the dot as he'd have bagged the lion by then.

'Sorry, Paul,' she apologized. 'I did try to explain you might have other visits booked as well but he hung up on me.'

I reassured her that I'd do my best to get there on time and, no, I wasn't going to treat a real lion.

When I arrived the following morning, the major was deadheading roses, a battalion of which were planted in formal ranks round the edge of the front lawn. I could picture him parading up and down, inspecting each one for the merest suspicion of black spot, the slightest touch of mildew. He swung his arm out and twisted his wrist to give an exaggerated look at his watch as I climbed out of the car. I'd already noted the time. 11.35.

'I've just phoned the surgery,' he said, snapping his secateurs in the air. 'I was wondering where you'd got to.' The glare from the hooded eyes and the waving secateurs suggested I could be next in line for deadheading.

I wasn't going to apologize for being five minutes late, so with my black bag in one hand, cat-catcher and leather gauntlets in the other, I walked up the path and said, 'You've got the cat then?'

'It's all going according to plan. Leo's in the greenhouse.' The major winced as he picked up his stick and proceeded to hobble towards the building. 'Damned leg's playing up today. 'Fraid I won't be of much help.' Beryl had told me about his leg. Apparently the major liked people to think it was the result of having been gored by a rhino. But her receptionist friend from the health centre had let it slip that it was nothing more than a touch of arthritis brought on by old age.

As we rounded the corner of the cottage, I noticed a trail of string hanging from the kitchen window and fastened to the door of the greenhouse.

Major Fitzherbert stopped to explain. 'When I was sure Leo was inside the greenhouse, I pulled the door shut from the kitchen. Clever, eh?'

'Er, good idea but—' I'd just side-stepped a large plate of congealing chicken casserole and looked down at it.

The major butted in, 'You can forget that malarky. I guess Leo could smell the tablets in it.' There was a hint of pride in his voice.

'You mean to say—'

'He didn't take them.'

He saw my mouth drop open. 'Nope. Not one scrap,' he added, giving me one of his penetrating stares. 'It doesn't bother you, does it? With that contraption of yours you can still catch him.' He waved at my cat-catcher.

'Well … yes … I can … but it might have been easier if he'd been a bit sleepy.' I put down my equipment. As the panes were misted up, I gingerly slid open the greenhouse door a fraction and peeped in. The cat was nowhere to be seen. I made the mistake of asking, 'You sure he's in there?'

'Good grief, laddie. Of course he is. I was the one who trapped him. Saw him go in with my own eyes.' The major's caterpillar eyebrows met and wiggled. 'No doubt he's in there just waiting to pounce.' He emphasized the word 'pounce' with such gruffness that I jumped – something he was quick to notice. 'Not scared are you?'

'No … no … not at all,' I lied, shaking my head, my innards already turning to jelly at the prospects ahead.

'Good. Wouldn't like to think you were a namby-pamby.'

'But as Leo didn't take the tablets, we may well have quite a fight on our hands.' My hands actually, I thought miserably. 'And if he starts to dash around you may find a lot of your plants get damaged.'

The major seemed unperturbed. 'Can't be helped. Leo's got a large gash on his back. It needs attention.' He stepped forward and thrust his face in mine. 'And you're going to give it. Right?'

I felt like jumping to attention with a smart salute. Instead I nodded and reached down for the cat-catcher. This consisted of a hollow metal tube threaded with a strong loop of cord which, if one was lucky – there that word again – one could lasso over a cat's head and pull tight to restrain the animal. Well, that was the theory. I had yet to put it into practice.

The major gave a derisive snort. 'Don't hold out much hope for that contraption.'

'It's all we have.'

'You should dart him.' He levelled two fingers like the barrel of a pistol at me. 'Bang. Over he goes. No problem.'

I bit my tongue, fighting back the urge to remind Major Fitzherbert that Leo was not a lion but a feral cat of ordinary proportions – least I assumed that to be the case as I had yet to set eyes on the wretched creature. Besides which I wasn't a good shot. My pub-playing-darts was proof of that. So even if we did have a dart gun, it would still have been a hit-or-miss affair. More miss than hit with me, more likely to anaesthetize a potted palm rather than Leo.

Clutching the cat-catcher in one hand, I slipped into the greenhouse to be immediately assailed by a wall of hot, humid air. I felt the sweat sprout from my upper lip while my armpits dripped.

There was a sharp rap on the glass, the blurred face of the major beyond the condensation. 'Seen him yet?' he demanded.

'No. Not so far.' I slowly crunched down the central path, nervously glancing from left to right. The towering mass of greenery surrounding me was so dense it could have hidden a posse of pussies. The dark green leaves of a giant philodendron rustled. I paused and then tiptoed forward. A flash of black slipped behind a palm. With the pole starting to slide through my greasy fingers, I stopped again and was just wiping my palms on my trousers when Leo padded into view framed in a shaft of sunlight. He was a magnificent tom, broad headed with scarred twisted ears. He stopped when he saw me. Large green eyes, the pupils mere slits, stared at me, oozing defiance. With a loud, rattling hiss, he arched his back. The 'Puss ... Puss....' I was about to utter faded on my lips. I could see the wound Major Fitzherbert had been concerned about – a jagged lump of skin torn from the cat's right shoulder blade. As I took a step closer, Leo melted behind a clump of bamboo.

'Blast you,' I muttered, as I continued to move forward, advancing on the bamboo, the cat-catcher held out in front of me. Suddenly a loud snarl rent the air. There was a flash of black. I ducked as Leo hurled himself over my shoulder, his claws slicing through my jacket as he scrabbled past my head. I swung round, the cat catcher veering in a wide circle, the noose slicing across an adjacent potting bench, scooping out a tray of fuschia cuttings, sending them spinning into the air and pattering onto the wall of the greenhouse like a hail of bullets.

There was another rap on the glass. 'What the hell's going on in there?'

'It's just Leo. He's proving a bit difficult to catch.'

There was a chuckle. 'That sounds like my Leo. Bit of a tearaway if ever there was one.'

I couldn't agree more. My torn jacket was testimony to that.

Two crushed cinerarias, a squashed begonia and three severed azaleas later, I managed to snare Leo amid a torrent of hisses and spits.

Only then did the major venture in brandishing his stick triumphantly. 'Jolly good show,' he bellowed. 'Reminds me of when I bagged my first lion.' He placed a restraining foot on Leo's squirming back as instructed, while I pumped in the anaesthetic injection I'd already drawn up. I breathed a sigh of relief as Leo's writhings slowly subsided and he slumped into unconsciousness.

The major didn't comment on the piles of uprooted seedlings on the potting bench; he merely swept them to one side to clear a space.

'So let's have him up,' he declared enthusiastically, seeming to be energized by the heat while I felt more and more like a limp lettuce.

Freeing Leo's inert body from the noose, I pulled him up onto the bench top. The major pushed me aside in his eagerness to look at the wound. 'Ah. Ah. Just as I thought. It's fly-blown. See?' He poked a finger and thumb in the wound and held up a wriggling white maggot. 'Saw it once in a leopard I shot. It ruined the pelt.'

I fetched my black bag and began cleaning up the torn skin, snipping back the matted hair, wiping away the yellow ooze and dipping a pair of tweezers into the seething mass of grubs, to pick them out one by one.

'Drop them in there,' instructed the major, pointing to an empty seed tray. 'Twenty four,' he said, when I'd finished. 'Pity I don't still fish.' He shuffled the tray from side to side watching the maggots roll round and round. 'Just think,' he mused. 'Poor old Leo walking round with that little lot squirming around under his skin. Just proves what a tough little blighter he is.' As he spoke, he lifted up the cat's tail and peered between his legs. 'By jove. What whoppers. Bet he's the talk of the town amongst the ladies around here.'

I paused midway through dusting the wound with anti-parastic powder. 'Do you want me to castrate him while he's under?'

'What ... and turn him into a poofter? No way.'

With the wound cleaned and powdered, I gave Leo a long-acting shot of penicillin. 'I'm afraid the area's too large to stitch. We'll just have to leave it to granulate over.'

'Then I'll keep him confined to barracks,' declared the major. 'He'll stay in the greenhouse.'

Throughout the following week, Beryl was inundated with progress reports on Leo: the times he was fed; the state of the wound; his daily movements within the greenhouse. Lucy came back from the local delicatessen to inform me a special order had been placed by Major Fitzherbert for daily supplies of tuna, smoked salmon and herring mops. I also heard that his friends were being coerced into coming round to see the invalid and watch the major stalk in to feed him. 'Leo's the talk of the town,' said Lucy. 'Well, at least of Gainsborough Drive. And apparently they're doing a feature on him in the *Westcott Gazette*.'

What next I wondered. Southern TV? National coverage? Then suddenly all went quiet. No further news.

'No, he hasn't phoned for the last couple of days,' Beryl told me.

So I assumed all was well and that the wound had healed. No doubt Leo was back in the wild stalking the Downs. So it was purely by accident that I bumped into the major in the local supermarket when I was trying to decide on which ready-meal to take back to Mrs Paget's.

I had to ask. 'So how's Leo?'

'Well ... he's OK,' whispered the major, a measure of doubt in his voice. 'Only....' He faltered, looking round as if afraid of being overheard before beckoning me across to a less crowded spot by the freezer compartment. 'Between you and me, he seems to have gone a bit soft in the head.'

'Really? In what way?'

'Well, he's just not the same cat. Lost all that wildness. Always indoors now, forever purring round my ankles, looking for his next bowl of fresh fish.' The hooded blue eyes gave me one of their customary stares. But there was a twinkle in them, a hint of humour. 'I don't consider him a Leo any more. So I've renamed him.'

He gave another surreptitious look round before continuing, 'He's now called Cuddles.' With that, he gave a short harrumph, threw a couple of packs of frozen coley in his basket and hobbled off.

I gave a sigh of relief. It was fortunate I'd been able treat the cat. With any luck there wouldn't be a repeat performance. I reached out to tap a shelf. It was metal.

Damn! Now where was a wooden one?

Chapter 4

One Friday evening, surgery was particularly hectic.

Beryl apologized several times as I came through from my consulting-room only to find she'd squeezed in yet another person to see. Even with the newly extended time I was allowed in Mrs Paget's kitchen, hopes of ever getting back there to pop a lasagne or lamb stew-with-dumplings-for-one in the microwave rapidly faded. Crystal was away for the day – some advanced orthopaedics course. No doubt she'd return brimming with new techniques for joint surgery putting my nose well and truly out of it – joint-wise that is.

Eric was on duty with me. He was just as busy, with a constant stream in and out of his consulting-room. When the last animal was ushered out, Eric rolled into the office with far less customary bounce than usual and collapsed in a chair like a crumpled carrier bag.

'Streuth,' he declared, mopping his glistening forehead with a swab. 'What did we do to deserve that I wonder? Seemed like all of Westcott's pets suddenly decided to take a sickie.' He gave me a rueful grin. 'Still you coped OK did you?'

'Just about,' I replied, my stomach giving a loud rumble, reminding me it was looking for its ready-meal. Some hope. It was way past 7.30. Mrs Paget's kitchen would now be out-of-bounds.

'Fancy a quick jar?' he added. 'Mandy's taking the phone tonight. I'll tell her we're just across the road. She knows I'm on duty so she can get me on my mobile. Come on. We both need to unwind a bit.' He paused and gave me an encouraging look, one eyebrow curled. 'So what do you say?'

Five minutes later saw us sitting round a table in the Woolpack, each with a lager and a large Cornish pasty in front of us. The pub was situated a stone's throw from Prospect House on the other side of what was euphemistically called the Green. 'Green' was a bit of a misnomer for this worn patch of parkland, now parched and burnt brown with the blistering summer we were having, coupled with a hosepipe ban – the only sprinkling it was getting was from the dogs peeing on it. The Green was bordered on three sides by busy roads, constantly choked with traffic, so taking the air usually meant taking in lungfuls of fumes. The Woolpack's sign of a shepherd with a lamb slung over his shoulder harked back to the days when sheep still grazed at its front door and shepherds still ploughed in for their ploughman's. Now the only reference to 'shepherds' was with the 'pie' on the menu board and any mention of 'fleece' was in reference to the exorbitant bar prices.

Eric took a hearty swig of his lager and wiped his lips free of foam before saying, 'So, Paul. You've settled in, eh?'

I too took a measured mouthful before attempting to reply. 'Er ... yes ... fine.' I wasn't sure how to play this. As far as I could judge, Eric seemed a very affable sort of guy; quite down-to-earth; no airs or graces; ready to call a spade a spade. So if I had any grumbles, he'd be prepared to listen. But to act on them? There I wasn't so sure. After all, he was married to Crystal, and she ruled the roost at Prospect House as far as I could see –both professionally and, no doubt, privately. I couldn't imagine anything ever happening without her say-so. Sharpe by name and sharp by nature. No blunt knives in her drawers.

'So there's nothing on your mind? Nothing you'd like to discuss?'

'Well....' I took another sip. Come on Paul. You don't need Dutch courage. Spit it out. So I did. 'When's the practice cottage likely to become available?'

'Ah yes. Willow Wren. Sorry about that. I know it was promised you, but there's been a bit of a problem with the current tenant. Crystal's sorting it out. Best to have a word with her about it.'

So I'd be a little longer in Mrs Paget's hands, I thought. Oh well. I'd just have to grit my teeth. I only wished that chihuahua of hers would grit his and stop going for my ankles whenever I stepped out of my room.

Talking of teeth, I was suddenly conscious of some rather large gnashers that were being exposed at a level with my knee. They belonged to a very large, very fat, very friendly yellow Labrador who was grinning at me, lips curled back exposing a fine set of canines while her eyes were fixated on the pasty from which I was just about to take a bite.

'Well hello, Peggy,' exclaimed Eric, with exaggerated enthusiasm, leaning across to vigorously fondle her ears, obviously thankful for the distraction. She sat down heavily and raised a paw which Eric shook. 'There's my girl.'

Peggy's grin seemed to expand, her lips curling back even more.

Eric turned to me. 'It's her way of asking for titbits.'

Perhaps I should practise her technique in order to get the practice cottage I thought. Actually I quite liked the idea of kneeling in front of Crystal with my tail wagging. Meanwhile it was just grin and bear it for me. 'Doesn't look as if she needs any,' I said.

Peggy was huge. Obese. She sat there, on fat, bulging haunches, one back leg splayed out, exposing rolls of belly fat.

'Couldn't agree more. But it's her party piece. The grinning. Isn't it, girl?' Eric broke off a portion of his pasty and offered it to her. It was snatched with alacrity and barely touched the sides of her throat as it was swallowed. Another grin followed.

'You shouldn't be doing that, Eric,' said a voice over my shoulder. 'You're always telling me she should be on a diet.'

'I know … I know,' he said, hastily dropping the next bit of pasty he'd intended giving Peggy and looking up.

I twisted in my seat to find a tall, heavily built woman standing behind me with a tray in her hand. She had frizzy blonde hair with dark roots and broad arched brows like drawn bows from under which she was shooting arrow-like looks at Eric.

'And you a vet.' The woman tutted but in an amiable way.

She levered herself round our table. Not an easy task as space was limited and amply filled by her ample posterior. She looked at me. 'Your friend here is always telling me I should get some weight off.'

For a moment I thought she was referring to herself as the broad hips, thighs, biceps and chest highlighted by the pink T-shirt and contour-hugging cotton trousers she was wearing suggested calorie counts didn't figure in her life, and if they did then she was a poor mathematician.

But I realized she was referring to Peggy when she bent over to give the Labrador a pat as Eric introduced her – Brenda. She and her husband, Bernie, I was told, were the Woolpack's proprietors.

'Fat chance of you losing weight, eh Peggy?' Brenda went on to say. 'Not with the likes of Eric slipping you titbits.'

Fat chance. Hmm. An unfortunate choice of words I thought in the circumstances.

But it was chance, fat or otherwise, that got me landed with Peggy's pounds not three days later.

Beryl was in one of her black moods, dress-wise and mentally. As usual she was wearing black, her raven hair stiff with lacquer. She clicked her scarlet nails over the computer keyboard, muttering softly to herself like a Macbeth witch incanting spells over a steaming cauldron. Black magic filled the air – and not of the chocolate box variety. Nothing sweet about Beryl today.

My cheery 'Good morning, Beryl' was met with a sour look and a downcast eye – while her glass one swivelled to the ceiling.

'You've a visit booked later this morning,' she said gruffly. Bubble … bubble … Beryl and trouble.

I raised an eyebrow which she was quick to spot.

'Couldn't get them to come in. Besides it's only over the road. The Woolpack.' The disapproval slurped out. I knew from Eric that though she was not teetotal – a port and lemon went down very nicely thank you, especially if someone else was paying for it – she showed her disapproval at the liquid refreshment that Eric occasionally indulged in at lunchtimes over at the Woolpack. He'd once returned reeking of alcohol. 'Just as well you're not operating this afternoon,' she'd said. 'You could anaesthetize a great Dane with one breath.'

'Is it Peggy?' I asked.

She gave a curt nod. 'The Adams's Labrador. Yes. She's off her legs and they can't move her. Not surprised. She's so overweight. Takes after her owners.' Stir … stir….

Mind you, she was right about the Adamses.

Bernie Adams introduced himself when I eventually got over to the pub. He was as massive as his wife, big, beefy, barrel-chested, with a flat pan of a face and large protruding ears that wouldn't have looked out of place on a Toby Jug. He was 'ale and hearty in every sense. A typical mine host.

'Brenda's upstairs with Peggy now,' he said, ushering me in through the pub's bar. The stairs were steep and narrow but only one flight; so no scaling of Everest, but to judge from the shortness of breath it provoked in Bernie I half expected a Sherpa guide and a cylinder of oxygen to be waiting on the landing. How on earth did Peggy, with all her pounds, manage to climb up and down?

She was lying stretched out on the kitchen floor, Brenda sitting squashed alongside in the narrow galley, wedged between the dog and a washing-machine. I put my black bag down on the work-top and crouched down by Peggy's head. Her lips curled back in their customary grin and her tail thumped on the vinyl, but there was no attempt to get up.

'Now, now, Peggy my girl. No need to worry.' I gave the Labrador a gentle pat on the head as Bernie leaned over me, his ears jiggling with anxiety 'We just need to find out what's wrong with you.' I levered myself up in the confined space. 'Now, Bernie, if you could just move back a bit. And you, Brenda, I just need to squeeze past.'

'OK, yes ... right.' Brenda struggled to her feet. There was much grunting and shifting of flesh as I squeezed myself between the lumbering Adamses feeling that at any minute I might be pulped before I managed to slip through, stepping over the dog to sink down over her hind quarters. I felt as if I'd just been swimming with a pod of whales especially when Brenda began to blubber, her shoulders heaving, asking if Peggy was going to be all right.

I elicited from Bernie that Peggy had been fine the night before and that they'd found her like this when they'd surfaced this morning. Moby Dick swam before my eyes as the words spouted from him. I quickly turned my attention to Peggy in an attempt to fathom out what was wrong with her. Poor dog was subjected to much prodding, pummelling and poking. A right hind here. A left hind there. Up a bit. Down a bit. Rotated both around a bit. It was a hokey-kokey of an examination throughout which Peggy just lay there, grinning. No grunt of pain. No squeal. Nothing. This wasn't what it was all about. I needed a diagnosis.

I began to panic – the situation was turning into a dog's dinner. It was hot, the flat an oven. The three of us gleaming like roasted potatoes with a Yorkshire pudding that had failed to rise at our feet.

'Let's try getting her to stand,' I said. No mean task considering the confines within which we were working.

Much huffing and puffing and further large movements of flesh followed – the Adamses' flesh in particular.

And a fat lot of good it did too.

We got Peggy onto her feet only for her to skid on the vinyl floor, her claws skittering in all directions; then down she sank again.

'We need a less slippery surface,' I wailed – Flipper had nothing on the way I was beginning to feel. 'Your lounge perhaps?'

Bernie shook his head. 'No better in there. It's got wooden floors.'

'Bedroom?'

'The same.'

I felt myself getting hotter and hotter. We had to do something. No way could the dog be left where she was, sprawled out like a lump of dough, loafing about on the kitchen floor.

Brenda butted in. 'Perhaps if we could get her down into the garden, that might get her moving. She loves sniffing round the tables looking for the odd dropped crisp. What do you think?'

Bernie snorted, harpooning her idea with one look. 'Just how do you think we'll get her down there. Crane?' He glowered at her. She glowered back. I could feel the heat rising between them. I felt I had to smother the tension before we had a volcanic eruption on our hands. I interrupted, 'A blanket.'

They both turned and stared at me. 'What?' they chorused.

'We could try a blanket as a sling to get her down the stairs.'

There was another snort from Bernie.

'Well it's worth a try,' said Brenda.

Bernie grimaced. ''Spose so,' he said, with distinct lack of conviction.

'Oh for goodness sake,' thundered Brenda, storming off to return moments later with a duvet cover. 'It's the best I can do,' she said apologetically, as she handed it across to me.

Once we had managed to lever Peggy onto the cover, we slid her out onto the landing and with me at the front, holding one end of the duvet cover, Bernie at the other, Peggy stretchered between us, we began the descent of the stairs. My fingers, tightly entwined in each corner of the cover, started to go numb. Any minute I thought Peggy would roll forward, knock me flying and pulverize me at the bottom, but we made it without anyone getting puréed in the process.

In the garden we hoisted Peggy to her feet again. This time she remained standing for nearly a minute, her hindlegs trembling violently, her sides like bellows, heaving with the exertion. Then she dropped, crashing onto the concrete in a mass of quivering flesh.

I began to despair.

'Look, I've an idea,' said Brenda. 'Just wait here a minute.'

'Well we're hardly likely to go anywhere,' muttered Bernie, giving her another dark look.

She returned waving a packet of crisps at us. 'They're Peggy's favourite. Smoky bacon.' She took one out and held it in front of the dog's nose. There was the sharp snap of jaws as the crisp disappeared in one doggy gulp. 'Nothing wrong with your appetite, girl,' she said, dangling another crisp just out of reach. Peggy grizzled and gave one of her lopsided grins, straining her neck forward, but she stayed splayed out, trembling.

'You know, it could be something quite simple like cramp,' I said, kneeling down next to Peggy's quivering hindquarters. I began to knead the muscles in her right thigh. After a few minutes I switched to her left leg. Peggy lay there, sighing, seeming to relish the pummelling.

'Right. Let's get her on her pins again,' I finally declared.

With no messing about, Peggy suddenly found herself yanked into a standing position with Brenda flourishing the crisp packet in front of her. 'Come on, sweetie. Have another crisp.'

'If you want one, you'll bloody well have to go and get it or else,' growled Bernie, his voice full of menace. The grin on Peggy's lips evaporated. She licked her lips. 'Well, go on then. Move yourself, you great fat mutt.' He raised his foot. 'Move.'

Peggy flinched and swayed like a rocking horse off its rockers; gave one tentative step forward; then waddled up to Brenda and buried her head in the crisp packet.

'See. Just needed a bit of persuasion,' said Bernie, as Peggy rapidly hoovered out the contents of the crisp packet and looked round for more.

Diet time for you, matey, I thought. A low calorie diet. No titbits. And weigh-ins on the platform scales at Prospect House.

Several weeks passed but the drop in weight I was looking for just didn't happen.

I complained to Bernie, 'Are you sure you're being strict about her diet?'

'Absolutely,' he declared. 'See here.' He showed me a booklet in which there were neat columns headed by days of the week, below which the types of food and amounts given were itemized.

Yet still Peggy's girth refused to shrink. Bernie and Brenda's enthusiasm for the exercise, or rather Peggy's lack of it, began to wane. The weekly weigh-ins became erratic. Consultations missed. Excuses made.

*

It must have been a couple of months later when Eric and I were again over at the Woolpack after yet another hectic Friday evening surgery.

Bernie was quick to apologize as Eric ordered a couple of lagers. 'Sorry. We've let things slip a bit,' he confessed. 'Being summer and all that. We're just so busy.'

'What was that all about?' queried Eric, as we settled at a table.

'See for yourself,' I replied, as Peggy waddled into view from behind the bar and came over to Eric with the usual lopsided grin on her face.

'Hello, fatso,' he said, reaching down to give her ears a tickle. 'Exactly,' I said. 'She's supposed to have been on a diet and lost weight.'

'Fighting a losing battle I'd say.'

Peggy shuffled off in search of customers willing to hand over a crisp or peanut in return for a sloppy grin of thanks. There were plenty on hand. I watched as another mouthful of calories was swallowed.

'You need a new strategy,' added Eric, downing his lager. 'Let's give it some thought. Drink up and I'll get another round in.'

By the time we'd finished our second pint we'd come up with a plan. A good plan. Excellent. Guaranteed to fight the flab. By our third pint we decided we'd write it up in the *Veterinary Record*. A stunning study. Well researched. By our fourth a doctorate in obesity was ours for the taking. Atkins Diet? Eat your heart out.

I made the mistake of mentioning the plan Eric and I had concocted to Mandy the next morning.

'I can't see it working, myself,' she said, her pinched lips and cold manner far more effective in sobering me up than the Alka-Seltzers I'd taken first thing.

'Really?'

'Really,' she echoed with a dismissive sniff.

Lucy, who had been folding vetbeds at the back of the ward intervened. 'Surely it would be worth a try. If it didn't work ... well ... nothing's lost.'

I saw Mandy check herself. 'It's not for me to say, of course,' she finally said, her eyes flicking from me to Lucy. If looks could kill, Lucy would have instantly become dead meat. Not for the first time I felt the tension between them.

She promptly contradicted what she'd just said by adding, 'But there's better things we could do with our time.' Her plum-coloured eyes continued to bore into Lucy as if trying to goad her into a rebuke. She glanced across at the stack of feed bowls waiting to be washed. The inference was obvious. I saw Lucy redden and her freckled nose twitch.

'I actually agree with Lucy,' I decided to say and watched – with delight I must confess – at how rapidly Mandy's face went pale save for two hectic blotches on each cheek. Now, now, Paul. Naughty boy. You should stay out of all this. But I felt the plan Eric and I had formulated the evening before had some merit – it had not been just the drink talking – and so was grateful of Lucy's support.

In fact, thanks to her the plan actually got put into practice.

She volunteered to find out the calorie content of anything that Peggy was likely to be offered as titbits in the pub; and within twenty-four hours had come up with a list of the calories in a crisp, peanut, a chip, a variety of chocolate bars and portions of sandwiches and pasties.

'It's a bit hit and miss,' she confessed.

'That's not a problem,' I said. 'It's just to give people a guide.'

When I gave Bernie the list his raised eyebrows said it all. He handed it to Brenda. 'What do you think?'

'Well I suppose it's worth a try. Nothing ventured nothing gained.'

Except more pounds on Peggy I thought.

So we went ahead. Anyone caught giving Peggy a titbit had to put a calorie fine in a charity box displayed prominently in the bar. The amount of the fine was proportional to the estimated number of calories in the titbit.

Bernie told me later that one teenager, his tongue loosened by too many alcopops, asked whether the slim-in was for Peggy or Brenda and nearly got a pasty in his face as a result. 'And he wasn't the first to crack that joke,' Bernie said. 'Brenda's getting quite touchy about it all.'

As part-instigator of the plan I decided it would be wise to steer clear of the Woolpack for a while. Just to be on the safe side. If Brenda was getting sensitive about her own weight then I didn't want to rub it in by asking about Peggy's and get a pasty in my face for my efforts.

*

But the finish of another hectic Friday surgery a few weeks later had me over there, cajoled by Eric – just for a quick jar. Or two.

'You do realize this is becoming a bit of a habit,' I said.

'What the heck. You need to wind down a bit. Relax,' he replied. No mention was made of whether Crystal approved or not. I decided it was best not to ask.

The list and charity box had disappeared. Hmm ... not a good sign, I thought uneasily. Bernie seemed cheerful enough, though did I detect a slight hollowness in his bonhomie? But I had to ask the question.

'So how did it go?'

'Well ... it sort of worked,' he said, pulling a face as he pulled our pints.

'Come on, Bernie. What do you mean "sort of"?' said Eric.

Bernie shrugged. 'As soon as the regulars realized how much it was costing them in calorie fines, the titbits stopped.'

'Well, there you are then. Our plan worked. It must have helped Peggy's diet.'

Bernie flapped his jug ears and looked doubtful. 'Well, I tell you, Peggy's not half the dog she used to be.'

I choked on my lager. What was he on about? Not half the dog? Had something gone wrong? Had the dieting upset her?

'See for yourself,' said Bernie, raising the bar flap. Unable to control himself any longer, he burst out laughing as Peggy trotted through, the half-dog he'd mentioned. Streamlined, fit, half the weight she used to be.

'She looks fantastic,' I said. 'Well done. I bet Brenda's pleased.'

'In more ways than one,' said Bernie still chuckling. He pointed a finger over my shoulder.

'Good lord,' spluttered Eric. 'Who'd have thought....'

I spun round to find Brenda, hands on hips, in a figure-hugging black dress, the figure it hugged being a shadow of its former self. She twisted her hips and gave a little twirl.

'Good eh?' she said. She went on to explain, 'Lucy was a great help. She lent me all the books on calorie control and seemed to know quite a bit about dieting. I thought it was worth a go. So, what do you think? Do you approve?'

There was a loud woof from Peggy.

'Sorry,' added Brenda. 'I should have included Peggy. Seeing that she was able to lose so many pounds I didn't see why I couldn't do the same.'

Except you weren't snuffling round customers eagerly looking for titbits. The thought made me smile. I looked down at Peggy. Was she thinking the same? Her lopsided grin suggested she did.

Chapter 5

It was amazing how those first few weeks at Prospect House flew by. Weeks in which I rarely met up with Crystal for more than a brief exchange of pleasantries. No doubt my tête-à-têtes with Eric filtered back to her: though no action had yet been taken regards the practice cottage. I was kept in the picture as to her movements – Beryl made sure of that. Each day she referred to Crystal's list of visits to those 'special clients', and Mandy made sure Tuesdays were kept sacrosanct for Crystal's ops – orthopaedic work in particular. It seemed our Dr Sharpe was destined to take the high road through the practice while I took the much humbler track that wound through the routine spays, castrates, dentals and more run-of-the-mill consultations.

So it was with some surprise that she stopped me in the corridor a few days before the summer Bank Holiday.

'Paul, I've been meaning to have a word,' she said, flashing me one of her perfect smiles – no overshot jaw or crooked teeth for her. 'Have you a moment?' Though a question, it didn't require an answer. If asked for a moment from Crystal, you had to spare it whether or not there were several anal glands waiting to be expressed in the waiting room. A well-manicured, unvarnished nail pointed to the office. 'Shall we?'

With the door closed, Crystal gestured to a chair. I sat down while she leaned against the desk, a hand to each side, lightly grasping the edge. She looked immaculate as always. Her pale-cream linen suit uncreased. How she managed that I couldn't fathom as anything linen I wore very rapidly took on the look of a wrung-out dishcloth. 'So, Paul. You're finding the job interesting?' Her fingers strummed lightly.

'Well, yes,' I replied, wondering where this was leading.

'And you're managing to cope with the workload?'

'It's a bit hectic at times. But no more than I expected.'

'And no other problems?'

I shook my head. There was the question of the night duties and weekend rotas unevenly shared. No practice accommodation. The endless routine ops. But I was sure Crystal didn't want to hear that.

'Good. Good.' Crystal fiddled with the gold band on her left wrist, twisting it round and round.

'The Bank Holiday weekend's coming up.'

I nodded.

'And you're on duty.'

No surprise there. I'd been told weeks back that I'd be on call. Crystal and Eric were off on a city break to Venice.

'I'm sure you'll be able to cope.' There was a tinge of uncertainty in her voice which made the hairs on the nape of my neck tingle. Hello. I sensed something was afoot. And I was right when she went on, 'It's just that you could be called out by the Richardsons.' Crystal's steel-blue eyes glanced away from me and she momentarily chewed her bottom lip. 'It's just that they're a rather – how shall I put it – a rather demanding couple.'

Again, no surprise there. What clients of Crystal's weren't demanding? That's why they were Crystal's.

'They refuse to see anybody but me as a rule.' Two high spots of red appeared on Crystal's cheeks. 'Not even Eric. They fell out with him years back. Something to do with vaccinating their dogs,' she added, as if I required an explanation. 'Sorry. You're wondering where all this is leading.'

I gave a wan smile and shrugged my shoulders. Wherever it was leading it didn't bode well.

Crystal continued, 'Well, they own this horse. And they're absolutely potty about her. Quite over the top to be honest with you.' Again she paused. 'Problem is they put her to stud.'

I groaned inwardly praying not to hear what I suspected was coming next. But to no avail.

'She's due to foal this coming weekend.'

Damn. I just knew it. Crystal saw me wince.

'Sorry. It's just one of those things. Of course the Richardsons are in an absolute tizzy imagining all sorts of horrendous things that could go wrong. And they're very put out that I'm going to be away at such a crucial time. They even suggested I cancel my holiday and they'd reimburse me for it. Can you imagine?' She looked apologetically at me. 'I've tried to reassure them that they'll be in your capable hands should they experience any problems. Hopefully that situation won't arise.'

Crystal didn't sound at all convincing. Nor was I convinced.

'Has the pregnancy been going OK?'

'No problems so far. Though George Richardson's imagination's running wild. He keeps on about breech presentations, eversion of the womb, heart blocks ... you know the sort of thing.'

That was just it. I didn't know and the mere thought of them made my innards feel like they were everting let alone those of an expectant mare. 'I don't suppose they could be wrong about the timing,' I said.

Silly of me to suggest it. But then I was clutching at straws. Whole bales of straw ... stacks of them to be honest.

The look in Crystal's eyes said it all.

The Saturday of the Bank Holiday kept me busy what with the influx of visitors to Westcott swelling the usual run of injured or sick cats and dogs. There were a couple of road accident cases: and a dog with a fractured femur which, as Crystal was away, I pinned myself despite oblique suggestions from Mandy that I referred the case, and I was pleased with my efforts.

There was no word from the Richardsons. I began to convince myself that they'd got their dates wrong. Even so I warned Mandy, the duty nurse for that night, re the possibility of a foaling. So the clamour of Mrs Paget's phone in the early hours of Sunday morning came as no great surprise. And yes, it was Mandy.

'Sorry, Paul. But I've just had Mr Richardson on. They're worried about their horse, Clementine. They insist on speaking to you.' She gave me their number.

Mr Richardson must have been sitting on the phone as he answered it at the first ring. With panic in his voice he said: 'Clementine's started. We need help immediately before she dies.'

I could sense his agitation down the phone. It was infectious enough to make my hand start shaking. Get a grip, Paul, I muttered to myself as I promised to get over as soon as I could. I phoned Mandy back to tell her of my plans.

'By the way,' she said, 'Lucy told me to say she'd be happy to help out if you needed her.' There was a pause. 'I'll wake her up, shall I?'

It was said as if Mandy relished the thought of doing so. And probably did as there was still no love lost between the two of them. 'I'll get her to be outside the hospital in ten minutes' time then,' she added, when I agreed to her coming.

'Everything all right?' A voice echoed down from the landing as I put down the phone. Mrs Paget stood at the top of the stairs, her head festooned with pink curlers, a hand clasped to the collar of her nightie, the other pinning a growling Chico to her waist.

"I've got to go out on an emergency. Not sure when I'll be back.'

'Well, don't worry. Whatever time it is you can use the kitchen. We won't mind, will we, Chico?' Mrs Paget gave the dog a kiss on his head and stared intently down at me. 'Anything to help the nice young vet here.' She continued to study me, her puffy eyes glinting.

I was suddenly aware I was only in boxer shorts and, thanking her, dashed back into my room to get dressed.

Lucy was waiting by the gate as I drove the short distance up the road to Prospect House. She nipped in front of the headlights and slipped into the car. The denim jeans and yellow sweatshirt moulded to her elfin-like figure reminded me how attractive she was. But then I always did like the gamine type.

Crystal had left me directions of how to get to the Richardsons' place. 'Well, you never know,' she'd said, handing me the map she'd drawn. I gave the directions to Lucy while thanking her for offering to help out.

'No problem,' she said. 'I've always wanted to see a foaling.'

Hmm, I thought. Preferably one without any complications. I had an uncanny feeling this one was not going to be straightforward. Not by a long chalk.

The Richardsons' farm was the other side of the Downs, on the outskirts of a village called Ashton. If it hadn't been for Lucy's map reading, her studying the directions with the aid of a small pencil torch, I'd have missed the lane in the dark and overshot the entrance to the farm; but twenty minutes' drive from Prospect House found ourselves on the farm's gravel drive, my headlights picking out the tall, angular figure of George Richardson as he strode briskly towards us, his arms waving like windmills. Even though it was three o'clock in the morning, he was impeccably dressed in tweeds and polished boots.

'Over here,' he barked, and directed us into a stable-yard with another anxious twirling of his arms. 'Quick before we lose her.'

'Blimey. He's in a bit of a panic, isn't he?' murmured Lucy, as I braked sharply. He wasn't the only one. My chest felt as if a belfry of bats was trying to claw its way out of my chest. Flit ... flit ... flutter ... flutter.... I raced round to the boot of the car to yank out my smock, ropes, disinfectant and black bag.

'Let me bring those,' said Lucy.

'Er ... right ... fine,' I stuttered, before dashing after the shadowy figure of Mr Richardson as he marched across to a loose-box, one arm still above his head, his hand beckoning us. He turned as I caught up with him by the door. 'Could have a breech on our hands,' he declared, staring at me. Winged eyebrows gave him a questioning look. His eyes bored into me. Red-rimmed, they matched the salami-blotched colouring of his cheeks. His shoulders twitched up and down like a manic mannequin. 'You're...?

'Mitchell. Paul Mitchell. And this is Lucy.' I turned as she hurried up, her arms loaded with my gear.

George Richardson gave her a cursory glance before saying, 'My wife's with Clementine now. She's in great pain.'

The wife? I thought momentarily. No, of course, silly, the horse.

'Has she started foaling down yet?' I asked.

'No. But we think she's about to start any minute now. That's why we've called you out. You don't think we'd waste your time otherwise, would you?' George gave another shoulder twitch and shot me and then Lucy a querulous look, his winged eyebrows waving, as he paused, hand on the bolt that secured the lower half of the stable door. The loose-box itself was ablaze with light. He leaned over the door and shouted 'Hilary, Dr Sharpe's stand-in is here.'

I peered in. A middle-aged woman with a face, moist and white like the underside of a fillet of haddock, was pulling on a head collar, determinedly marching round a bay brown mare who was reluctantly shuffling through the paper bedding, a ball of it wrapped round each fetlock.

'There, there,' she crooned, stopping to whisper in the horse's ear. 'The vet's here to make you better.'

'I jolly well hope so,' said her husband, slamming the bolt back and ushering me in. 'Even if it's not Dr Sharpe.'

'I'll wait outside until you need me,' whispered Lucy.

Hilary's free hand shot out and clutched my arm in a vice-like grip. 'What is it? You look so worried. What's wrong with Clementine?'

I made a mental note to practise a reassuring smile in the mirror until I had it off pat. It seemed the Richardsons were in need of great dollops of reassurance. I had to exude confidence. Show my ability to deal with any problem foaling as if it was second nature to me – as if I'd dealt with hundreds of such cases even though this was my first.

'Nothing's wrong, Mrs Richardson. Clementine looks fine.' I smiled in what I hoped was a more confident manner.

'How can you tell?' said George gruffly. 'You haven't examined her yet.'

'He's just saying that to reassure us,' said his wife, letting go of me to reach across and claw her husband's arm.

I felt my smile falter. Oh dear. Seems I was overdoing the reassurance bit. But I meant what I'd said. Clementine did look fine. Despite my lack of experience, it was easy to see that the horse was in no sort of distress. There was no fidgeting; no tail swishing or stamping of feet. She looked completely relaxed. Which was more than could be said of the Richardsons – their twitchy movements, sweaty faces and wild eyes making them look as if they were the ones about to foal down at any minute.

Hilary turned to the mare and stroked her muzzle. 'She's got a pained look in her eyes. I can tell, you know. Look. Can't you see?' She yanked the horse's head round to me. Startled, the mare rolled her eyes, showing the whites, and then gave a loud snort and pulled away.

George stepped forward and ran a hand down Clementine's flank. 'Thought so. She feels warm. Shouldn't be surprised if she's running a temperature.'

'It's more likely to be the heat,' I murmured. It was the middle of the summer, a warm balmy July night and there were two electric fires strapped to the rafters, three bars glowing in each. 'It's really too hot in here. You should turn those off.' I pointed up at the fires.

'Are you quite sure?' said Hilary, her white face cut sharply by the questioning line of her vermilion lips. 'It's just that we didn't want the foal catching cold.'

'He won't, I assure you.'

'But—'

'If you're quite sure,' intervened George.

'Yes.'

'Well, l guess you should know what you're talking about.' George rubbed his bony hands together in time to his seesawing shoulders. 'No doubt you've attended plenty of foalings like this eh?'

I forced my reassuring smile and uttered 'Of course' just at the moment Clementine turned, looked at me and gave a loud snort. They say horses have finely tuned senses. Thank goodness they can't talk. 'Now I'm sure Clementine would like us to leave her in peace for awhile. Allow her to get on with things quietly.'

There was a joint intake of breath and simultaneous explosive gasps from both of the Richardsons.

'What, leave her without help?' queried George, jiggling his shoulders again.

I nodded.

'Are you quite sure?' said Hilary.

Oh dear. We were off again. This time my look said it all.

'Very well.' Reluctantly, Hilary unclipped the halter rope and allowed herself to be propelled outside with George close behind while I stayed in the loose-box.

I heard her address Lucy. 'I hope he knows what he's doing.'

'He's very competent,' she replied.

Good on you, Luce, I thought.

The Richardsons remained just outside of the stable door, fidgeting on the spot. I racked my brains for a means to get them away so as to give the mare a better chance to settle down.

'I think we might need some buckets of warm water,' I heard Lucy say.

'Do you?' asked George, peering in at me.

'Er … yes … it might be useful.'

'You go then,' said George looking at his wife. 'I'll stay in case I'm needed.' Hilary's face contorted with doubt, but after a few seconds' hesitation, she finally backed away and disappeared into the darkness.

I had another idea. 'It would be a great help if I could have some strong bits of wood to use as handles on the foaling ropes.'

Like his wife, doubt creased George's face, his winged eyebrows quivered. It was then that Clementine chose to neigh and swing her head round at her abdomen.

George pointed. 'There … look … something's wrong.'

'Please Mr Richardson … the handles.'

'What if something happens while I'm away?'

'It won't.'

'But you never know—'

'The handles, please.'

Clementine emitted another soft, deep neigh. George alternately jerked each shoulder up and down, a finger and thumb constantly running back and forth across his lips. 'Well. OK,' he mumbled, and, with a final shrug of his shoulders, he gradually edged back.

With a sigh of relief, I let myself out of the loose-box and switched off one of the two blinding fluorescent lights. 'That's better,' I murmured. 'Now come on, girl. Hurry up and get on with it. You're giving all of us the heebie-jeebies.'

Clementine blinked. Her eyes, enormous indigo pools, stared briefly at me.

'Do you think she's due then?' asked Lucy.

'By the way she's beginning to behave ... yes ... see?'

Clementine had started to circle slowly round the box, shuffling methodically through the paper bedding while dark patches of sweat pricked through the hair over her flanks and under her shoulders. After five circuits, she slowly sank into the bedding with a rattling sigh.

As if from nowhere, the Richardsons appeared. A bucket crashed in the yard as Hilary came rushing across crying, 'What's happening? What's happening?' closely followed by George waving a couple of short lengths of wood in the air. The commotion brought Clementine scrabbling to her feet. We were back to square one.

I looked at Lucy. 'We need to keep them away,' I seethed. But how?

'What about a cup of tea?' Lucy suggested, as George and Hilary ground to a halt in front of us.

Tut. Tut. Bad idea, Lucy.

'Tea?' they chorused looking at each other in amazement.

'How could we possibly think of tea at a time like this?' remonstrated Hilary, her voice shrill with anxiety.

'Well, Clementine won't settle down with us all here,' I said bluntly. 'She needs peace and quiet. So maybe a cup of tea is not such a bad idea.'

George's shoulders began to twitch again. He suddenly squared them and turned to his wife. 'Seems we aren't wanted,' he said, with a sniff. 'Best have that cuppa after all.' With a curt nod in our direction he pulled his wife towards the house.

'Sorry about that, Paul,' said Lucy, her freckled face full of concern.

'Don't be,' I said. 'It's done the trick. Got them out of our hair for a bit. Now let's hope Clementine gets on with things.'

We turned to watch the mare. She snatched a mouthful of hay from her hay-net and nervously chewed it, her teeth grinding. Then she emitted another groan and dropped to the ground. This time she stayed there; and with legs stretched out, began to strain.

"Hooray. At last,' I muttered, as I rolled up my sleeves, donned my smock and slipped quietly into the loose-box. Lucy followed and knelt down by the mare's head and gently stroked her neck.

Liberally smearing my right arm with lubricating jelly, I began a gentle examination of the mare's inside. Clementine gave a little grunt, raised her head and crossed and uncrossed her fetlocks. 'There … there….' I said. 'Steady on.' The words were as much for my benefit as they were for hers, but they seemed to steady her as she sank back with a sigh.

I gingerly probed deeper. The relief was enormous when I felt first one tiny fetlock, then another. My hand slid past them, waiting any minute to feel the foal's head in its natural position between the feet. Instead I felt two more hoofs slip through my fingers. I checked. Yes. Two more hoofs. A wave of panic flooded me.

'Damn,' I said.

'Problem?' whispered Lucy.

''Fraid so.'

'Everything OK?' George was back, leaning over the door, his wife's ghostly pale face alongside.

I cautiously slid my arm out and stood up, my guts churning and pinging, my legs shaking. 'Well, actually there is a problem.'

'Problem?' exclaimed Hilary, her mouth dropping open.

'What do you mean … problem?' added George, his salami cheeks blanching, his shoulders going into free fall. 'The foal's not dead is it?'

'No … no … it's not that bad.' I hesitated before saying the word. 'But it is a breech.' The word hung momentarily silent in the air between us before its meaning imploded on the Richardsons with predictable consequences.

'Oh my God,' screamed Hilary. She wrenched open the door, rushed in and pushing Lucy aside, flung herself down to cradle the mare's head in her lap. 'My poor, poor Clementine,' she moaned, tears streaming down her face. The mare was now beginning to strain more frequently; her flanks were black, darkly drenched with sweat; she groaned, clearly in pain.

George had followed Hilary in and was now standing right next to her all of a quiver, bristling with agitation. 'So what are you going to do about it? Call in an expert?'

Fighting to control my own jumpiness and keep my voice from sounding like an untuned banjo I answered, 'I'm going to give Clementine a sedative and then try a spinal anaesthetic.' Too late I realized I'd used the wrong words.

George pounced on them. 'Try? What do you mean try?' The wings on his eyebrows seemed to arch even higher as he spoke. 'I would assume you've done this sort of thing before.' He swung round to Lucy, eyes blazing. 'Well, hasn't he?'

She squared up to him as best she could. 'He'll be doing his best for Clementine. I assure you.'

I tried to put on a brave face, but my confidence was oozing out of my boots as fast as the fluids seeping from the mare's hindquarters. I had administered a spinal anaesthetic before. Once. And only once. And then that was under the watchful eye of our Professor of Surgery at Veterinary School. Here, with Clementine, I had no choice but to try. She had a foal facing the wrong way. That foal had to be turned round inside her womb before it could be delivered. And I couldn't turn the foal round with her straining. That had to be stopped, and the only way possible was by anaesthetizing the lower part of Clementine's body – blocking off the nerves to that area by giving an epidural.

By the look in Lucy's eyes, I realized she knew exactly how I felt. Petrified. It was pointless trying to persuade the Richardsons to leave me to it. They were far too concerned; to the extent they were almost shell shocked. Numbed. It at least allowed Lucy to shunt them into one corner without any objections being made while we got on with it.

'Lucy. You hold onto Clementine's head please. Make sure she doesn't move,' I instructed.

Hands shaking, I drew up a syringeful of anaesthetic. Now came the task of locating the exact spot where I had to inject it. Under the hawk-eyed gaze of the Richardsons I began pumping Clementine's tail up and down like I was attempting to draw water from a well. I felt her vertebra crack beneath my probing fingers. In my mind's eye I tried to recall the college lectures, those count-less anatomical diagrams, the pony skeleton with arrows pointing to where, at what angle and at what depth the needle had to be inserted without risk of it puncturing the spinal cord. The pumping of the tail was to help locate the exact spot. I kept on. Pumping. Pumping. Pumping. Finally, realizing I couldn't delay things any longer I sank the needle through the skin at what I thought was the correct place. Imagine my relief when a trickle of yellow fluid oozed out. Spinal fluid. Yippee! I'd hit the right spot. Attaching the syringe, I pushed down on the plunger and watched the dose of anaesthetic disappear.

'Phew,' I gasped, as I whipped out the needle and got to my feet. 'Least that's done.' I looked along Clementine's flanks now steaming with sweat and smiled at Lucy before turning to the Richardsons, still transfixed in the corner. 'Maybe a cup of tea while we wait for the anaesthetic to take effect?'

They obeyed without a murmur.

A fine drizzle had begun to sweep across the yard as the four of us returned from the house. Whether due to the trickle of water that ran down my neck or the thought of what still lay ahead, I began to shiver.

Clementine lay stretched out, quiet, motionless.

Hilary gasped, one hand flying to her mouth, the other catching at the sleeve of my smock. 'She's ... she's ... not dead, is she?'

Clementine lifted her head and whinnied.

Hilary let go of my sleeve with a sheepish look.

This time I allowed the Richardsons to cradle Clementine's head, while Lucy and I knelt down behind the mare where two tiny hoofs were poking out. I tied a rope round each of them and handed the ends to Lucy. No mention had been made of the need for wooden handles, or buckets of warm water for that matter. Best keep quiet about it, I reasoned.

'Keep some tension on those ropes, Lucy,' I said, as I once again slid my arm inside the mare's womb in an attempt to turn the foal round. As before, the other set of hoofs were just inside, and now that Clementine was no longer straining I was able to push them back. As I did so, I felt them float away from me. Hey. This was easier than expected. Then suddenly the floating stopped. I pushed on the legs. Nope. No movement. I pushed again. They didn't budge. Another push. Still they didn't shift. What on earth was stopping them? My heart thundered against my chest and I could feel trickles of sweat course down my cheeks, leaving a warm trail as they coalesced to drip from my chin.

'Not more problems, surely,' said an anxious voice, as George looked over at me.

I grunted. 'The foal's quite large. Proving a little difficult to turn.' I was now right up to my armpit and felt as if I was trapped inside, the folds of the womb like those of a collapsed tent, enveloping and hindering every movement of my arm.

Hilary suddenly yelled 'Clementine's suffocating.' Her cry made the mare jerk. My arm was violently squeezed, pinned to the wall of her pelvis, rotated and pulled until I thought it would be wrenched from its socket. I opened my mouth but forced back the scream that threatened to explode from my lungs. Lucy winced, grimacing in sympathy.

'Quiet, woman,' hissed George. 'It's just Clementine snoring.'

As the horse relaxed, the pressure on my arm subsided. But it was several minutes, with me stretched out in the bedding taking deep breaths, before I had sufficient strength and feeling in the arm to resume my attempt to swing the foal round. My fingers swam through the warm fluids, membranes yielding, sliding from me like layers of overcooked lasagne. Imagine the relief when my fingers finally bumped into the foal's melon-sized head. It was now just a matter of easing it towards me. Yeah. Right.

'Pull a little on the ropes, Lucy.'

She pulled. 'Enough?'

'A bit more.' I felt the foal's head float nearer. 'Bit more.' The back legs started to dip out of reach. Then they were gone. 'Done it,' I declared triumphantly. 'The foal's turned round.' I pulled my arm out and took one of the ropes from Lucy.

'We're going to start pulling quite hard,' I warned the Richardsons who, though still at Clementine's head, were both straining to see what was going on.

'Don't get too alarmed.'

'We should be so lucky,' murmured Lucy, wrapping her rope tightly round her palm.

'Right. Here we go. Heave.'

We both pulled together.

Clementine emitted a long, deep groan.

'You're hurting her,' cried Hilary.

'No, we're not,' I called out. 'She can't feel a thing.' In fact, with the epidural, Clementine couldn't even contract. Lucy and I were her labour. If we didn't pull, the foal wouldn't come out. So pull we did.

Pull. Pull. Pull. Slowly, the forelegs emerged, gleaming, steaming, covered in mucus. Then the head popped out, large, domed; to be rapidly followed by the long, brown sticky body of the colt. He plopped onto the bedding in a pool of yellow fluids.

Hilary jumped to her feet. 'Oh clever Clementine,' she cooed. 'You've produced a wonderful baby.'

'Yes, well done,' exclaimed George, echoing his wife's sentiments.

As for our part in the proceedings … Lucy and I just looked at each other and shrugged. At least Clementine seemed appreciative of our efforts. She gave a whicker of motherly concern and stretched round to give her son his first wash.

'Well,' said George, as we cleaned ourselves up in the kitchen. 'It seems congratulations are in order.' His shoulders smartly jigged up and down.

'Indeed yes,' added Hilary, her white face glowing, her thin lips curled back in a smile. 'We can't wait to tell Dr Sharpe.'

I squirmed with pleasure. It's not every day one receives compliments. So it's nice to get them when they come. 'Oh I'm sure that won't be necessary,' I murmured, hoping I said it with the right touch of modesty.

Hilary cut in, 'She'll be so pleased to hear how well behaved Clementine was. Such a model patient. It made your task so much easier I'm sure.' Her bland, milky eyes blinked at me. Soulless. What a slap down.

Dawn was breaking as we drove back over the Downs. The belt of rain had passed to leave a pencil of cloud scoring the pale eastern sky in a ribbon of pink. Below it the orb of the sun had began to edge up with promise of another hot day. It looked spectacular from the top of the Downs. So much so that despite my tiredness, I impulsively swerved into a lay-by overlooking the undulating fields which stretched down towards Westcott and the silver line of the sea beyond.

'Sorry. Hope you don't mind,' I said, turning to Lucy. 'It's just so beautiful.'

'I don't mind at all,' she replied, smiling shyly at me. 'In fact, I was rather hoping you would.'

We sat in companionable silence watching the sun rise over the far, grey-green line of hills. A giant ball of orange, the shimmering light from which gradually washed across the fields, painting in the yellow of the corn, the bright red of the poppies.

Without taking my eyes off the scene, I spoke. 'You know, I'm very pleased you came along tonight.'

'So am I,' said Lucy quietly.

Tentatively, I reached across and laid my hand lightly on hers. 'Then we must do it again.'

'I'd love to.'

As the sun continued to lift above the horizon, so did my spirits. Here it seemed was the dawn of a promising new day.

Chapter 6

When Crystal and Eric returned from their trip to Venice, I was immediately asked about the Richardsons. No surprise there. I'd sensed Crystal had been worried about the foaling and probably wondered whether I'd be up to the job. But then maybe that was just paranoia on my part. What was surprising was the warmth with which she responded to the fact that I'd delivered the foal by epidural.

'Let's hope George and Hilary appreciated what you did for them,' she said, eyeing her husband. 'Some people have been known to get on the wrong side of them all too easily.'

Eric reddened.

'I'll go and see what appointments Beryl's lined up for me,' he muttered, and shot out of the office.

Crystal shook her head, causing her copper curls to tremble as if each coil was charged with electricity. How I'd love to run my fingers through them and be shocked. I was given one of her dazzling smiles. Oh those cornflower-blue eyes. Yes, she was still my Julie Andrews. And yes, I could still skip for miles through meadows similarly flecked with cornflower blue, clasping that dainty hand with the gold bangle at the wrist. Providing she could keep up with me of course. After all she must be a good twenty years older than me.

'Paul. You all right?'

'Er, yes ... sorry. Miles away.' In Austria actually ... with the Von Trapp family ... but all too complicated to explain. Whatever, it seems I'd struck the right note with how I'd coped with the Richardsons. Either that or Crystal's holiday had put her in a particularly generous mood for suddenly the practice cottage – the one over in Ashton – was going to be at my disposal at the end of July.

'The tenancy finished then anyway,' said Beryl when I told her.

'So they'd want to make sure they got you in there as quickly as possible.'

Thanks, Beryl. You make a guy feel really good. She was standing in the doorway leading to the back garden having what she termed her 'in between' smokes, cigarette in her right hand, left hand, palm up, to catch the ash. Dreadful habit. But no one, it seemed, had been able to persuade her to stop smoking.

'Been doing it for fifty years and what harm has it done me?' she'd croaked when challenged, glaring out from a face full of wrinkles that would have done a prune proud.

She dragged on her cigarette and gazed out at the tired back lawn, worn from dog exercising, bare in patches from urine scald.

'You know, Mrs Paget will be sorry to lose you,' she confided. 'Cynthia's been a lonely woman since Henry walked out on her. Though she's got Chico of course.'

Ah, yes ... Chico. The ankle-biting chihuahua.

'But it's not the same,' she added, giving me a funny one-eyed stare. 'If you know what I mean.'

To judge from the look Mrs Paget had given me when she'd caught me in my boxer shorts I knew exactly what Beryl meant.

'She thinks a lot of you.'

I'm sure she did – especially out of my boxers. 'She let me have some freezer space,' I said, for want of something to say.

Beryl's good eye widened. 'Did she indeed. Then you were honoured.' She stepped onto the patio and tipped the ash in her palm over a wilting clump of lavender before stepping back in. 'Still you'll have all the freezer space you'll need over at Willow Wren. Especially if you're going to be on your own.' I was subjected to another glassy stare.

There. I knew it. She was fishing. In my first few days at Prospect House I'd told her I had a girlfriend in London – Sarah. I went up to see her a couple of times on my days off, but she was never keen to come down to Westcott-on-Sea. Maybe she thought it too fuddy-duddy for her. Whatever, distance in this case had made the heart grow weaker and we had gradually drifted apart with vague promises to keep in touch.

That was before the dawn of my relationship with Lucy, that magical moment on the Downs. We'd been discrete since, making sure nothing affected our working relationship. But people weren't daft – Beryl and Mandy in particular would have caught me looking at Lucy, a love-sick puppy dog expression on my face. And I'm sure the old totem drums would have been beating between Mrs Paget and Beryl, telling her of Lucy's visits to my lodgings. Originally, I had intended to ask Sarah down to share the practice cottage with me, assuming that we'd still be together. In the event, I found myself asking Lucy. There was no hesitation. 'I'd love to,' she'd said.

It did mean some reorganizing of rotas for night duty. But Mandy was surprisingly co-operative. Probably glad to get Lucy out of Prospect House. The two of them sharing the flat above the practice must have had its problems. Especially as they didn't seem to get on particularly well.

'Mustn't upset the nesting love birds,' she said. Sarcasm? Envy? There was a touch of something in the way she said it. But those damson eyes of hers gave nothing away.

It was decided Lucy would keep her room in the flat over Prospect House and stay there when it was her turn to take the phone at nights. Crystal and Eric didn't seem too bothered at us hitching up.

There was just the one moment, during a lapse of restraint, when Lucy was in the dispensary counting out some antibiotic pills for a patient and I was hunting for a can of flea spray, that the narrow confine of the dispensary proved too much for me as I squeezed past her; I found myself giving her a kiss at the moment Eric bounced in for some worm tablets. He grabbed a packet and backed out, muttering about a castration that ought to be done.

Willow Wren was a nineteenth-century, farm labourer's cottage, the end of a terrace of three, the other two having been made into one. It was next to what had been the village pond, surrounded by willows, hence its name. The pond had been filled in during the seventies and was now a cul-de-sac of houses dating from that period. The cottage still boasted a tall flint wall running down the length of a narrow back garden which, when we arrived, was a riot of brambles and overgrown shrubs. Clearly the previous tenants hadn't liked gardening.

The cottage itself was sweet. Whitewashed, red-tiled, a cat slide roof running down over the kitchen at the back. Inside, the wall between the two main rooms had been removed to make one large reception area, beamed with roughly hewn timbers and sporting a large brick-faced open fireplace with a honey-coloured oak bressummer. Up a steep flight of stairs there was a tiny landing with two doors leading off; one into a front bedroom with an uneven floor and sloping ceiling; the other through into a second bedroom off which was a bathroom with timbered walls and a view across the garden and beyond to the Downs. Very picturesque. I felt privileged to have been given this; all the more so as I had a pretty girl to live there with me. What more could I ask for? In the event there was going to be lots more. As I soon found out.

It was as we were picking our way through the jungle of the back garden, that we discovered, lurking under a welter of overgrown ramblers, a row of small aviaries backing onto the flint wall. There were three nesting sheds and four out-of-door flights, and considering the state of the rest of the garden they were all in remarkably good condition with no holes in their mesh.

'Hey this is some find,' said Lucy, gleefully. 'Couldn't be better.'

I caught her arm and swung her round to face me. Her eyes sparkled like dew on young acorns; the freckles on her nose danced.

'Now what's this all about?' I said drawing her close.

Her lips drew back in a wide grin.

'Come on. Out with it,' I added.

'It's just these aviaries....' She hesitated. 'They'll be perfect for waifs and strays.'

'Waifs and strays?' I echoed uneasily. 'What do you mean?' But I didn't have to ask. Lucy's life revolved around animals. They were her passion. So I might have guessed that when we moved into Willow Wren there would be an entourage of animals moving in with us. To start with it was small; a lame guinea pig and a rabbit that had lost an eye in a fight. But within weeks, the menagerie had grown. In one aviary twittered six budgerigars and two love birds; in another squeaked a hoard of guinea pigs; some ferrets and bantams appeared; while the cottage became home to three tabbies and a deaf Jack Russell called Nelson. To compound things, a goose turned up – but then she was my fault.

I arrived back after morning surgery one Saturday with a wicker basket. As I heaved it onto the kitchen table, there was a loud honk from inside. Lucy turned from chopping up some tomatoes and cucumber for lunch and said with a wry smile, 'Sounds like another addition to the family coming up.'

'Well, it's not exactly a pet,' I explained, beginning to unstrap the lid. 'I don't know if you remember that incident with one of Eric's clients: the Stockwell sisters' sheep?'

'Weren't they the ones that got savaged by a walker's dog? Yes I do remember. Hawkshill Farm. He had to go out and stitch several up.'

It had been three in fact; two others had to be put down.

'Well, this was a "thank you" present for him from the Stockwell sisters. Only he didn't want it. And has passed it on to us.'

As the lid of the basket creaked open, a long white neck uncurled from within.

I added, 'With five months to go before Christmas she should fatten up nicely.'

A large orange bill swung out, a steely-grey eye fixed me with a hard stare, and a loud hiss was spat in my direction. I felt almost obliged to say, 'Sorry. Didn't mean to offend you.'

In a flurry of snowy down and flaying webbed feet, the goose was scooped out of the basket. She ruffled her feathers, wagged her tail and promptly relieved herself on the floor before commencing a voyage of discovery, leaving a well demarcated trail behind her.

Ignoring the mess she was making, I enthusiastically explained that she was a variety of goose called an Embden.

'They make particularly good table birds,' I added, as our prospective Christmas dinner pecked at her reflection in the oven door.

'Have you thought where we'll keep her?' asked Lucy, her voice slightly on edge as she watched our posse of three cats glide into the kitchen, their eyes wide and gleaming as they spotted the young goose.

'I'm sure we can find somewhere.' I thought for a moment. 'There's a spare aviary, isn't there?'

Lucy shook her head. 'I've just put some more guinea pigs in there.'

'Well what about that old chicken coop?'

'I've got bantams in it.'

'The garden shed?'

'Where would the ferrets go?'

'No problem. They can be moved into the garage until Christmas. And don't look so worried.' I threw an arm round Lucy's shoulder and gave her a reassuring hug. 'I'll get her wings pinioned so there'll be no problem with her flying off.'

But I'd misinterpreted the concern in Lucy's eyes She was more worried about the hullabaloo that was imminent. The cats had encircled the goose and were crouched, ready to spring, tails twitching, whiskers quivering.

'If we're not careful....' she warned as the cats leapt forward. The goose let out an ear-splitting honk, flapped her wings vigorously and sailed into the air, skimming over the cats' heads to land with a deafening crash into the vegetable rack, its contents spilling out in all directions. The cats yowled and sprang for the back door just as Nelson tore in to start yapping furiously at an onion convinced it was the troublemaker. Lucy clapped her hands to her ears, hunched her shoulders and grimaced.

After the weekend, true to my word, I took the goose back to Prospect House to pinion her wings. Lucy refused to have anything to do with it, declaring it was cruel. Mandy, in her customary style, informed me there was a slot available just before lunchtime; as in the case of Miss McEwan's mynah, she was very efficient and had all the necessary instruments lined up waiting for me.

As the goose slipped into unconsciousness, she patted the bird's breast. 'I reckon there'll be enough there to feed a regiment come Christmas,' she said. 'Far more than you two could manage on your own.' She gave me one of her doe-eyed looks, her long dark eyelashes fluttering. If she was fishing for an invitation to Christmas lunch I chose to ignore it.

When I returned to Willow Wren with the goose, each plucked wing sported a neat row of stitches where the tip had been snipped off and the pimply skin edges sutured together. I carried the basket onto the patch of lawn we'd recently cleared at the back and tipped it on its side. The goose shuffled out with a couple of indignant honks before flapping her wings and with head stretched forward, skittered down the garden clearly expecting to get airborne. Instead, she plunged straight into the overgrown shrubbery at the end and disappeared from view. There was much crashing about and snapping of twigs before she re-emerged with a necklace of greenery draped round her neck and gave vent to a loud cackle before wobbling back up the lawn, bobbing her head up and down.

Lucy doubled up with laughter. 'A star turn if ever there was one,' she gasped, tears streaming down her face.

I agreed. 'A veritable Gertrude Lawrence.'

The name seemed apt. So Gertie she became.

By carefully rearranging Lucy's menagerie, I was able to find a home for Gertie in the potting shed. It proved an ideal shelter where she could be locked up at night to protect her from the local prowler – a fox with a taste for all things feathered. As for feeding her, this turned out easier than anticipated. Gertie liked eating grass. I disliked cutting it. So the lawn mower was abandoned in favour of the goose. As the grass grew so did her girth. Unfortunately, though the lawn was quite big, it did not quell Gertie's appetite to try pastures new; and we soon discovered Gertie had a knack of escaping that would have done the prisoners of Colditz proud.

The phone rang one Saturday afternoon when I was off duty. I had been in the process of trying to persuade Nelson that the vitamin tablet I was attempting to push down his throat in a lump of cheese was good for his health. I reached for the phone as he swallowed the cheese and spat out the pill. It was Joan Spencer, the postmistress who lived next door. She and her husband Doug, had introduced themselves when we'd first moved in, presenting us with a welcoming bouquet of sweet peas picked from their garden – a beautifully tended garden, bursting with blooms that put ours to shame.

'I'm sorry to trouble you,' she said, her voice full of agitation, 'but there seems to be a large white duck, or something, pecking at our pansies.'

Oh Lord. That white something just had to be Gertie. I tore round. And sure enough, there was Gertie on the edge of Mrs Spencer's patio now trying to decapitate a red plastic gnome. Seeing me advance up the path, she gave a cackle of greeting before turning to waddle into a bank of pink and white petunias. I headed her off but not before a neat row of dwarf marigolds had been trampled under web and a beakful of geraniums snatched.

Gertie's next port of call was the rectory across the other side of the lane. We were not church-goers and had yet to meet the local vicar of St Mary's church; Gertie made sure we did.

I answered the door to a tall, cadaverous man in a shiny grey suit with a dog collar that hung loosely round his scrawny neck. He had a long, lank head with muddy brown eyes and an upper lip that curled back over his teeth when he spoke. Very equine. I almost expected him to clasp his hands together and say 'Let us bray.'

Instead, in a sing-song reedy voice he said, 'I'm Revd Matthews. I do apologize for any intrusion that I might be causing when your time is precious, but have you perchance lost one of your ... er ... uhm ... flock?' He swayed towards me before rocking back on his heels. 'It's just that a goose has taken it upon herself to go for a paddle in our pond. I feel the nature of her exercise might be an upsetting element for the residents – my koi carp. If you understand what I mean.' Having finished his little sermon, his upper lip uncurled and settled into a wan smile.

I knew at once it had to be Gertie and, apologizing profusely, donned some wellingtons before accompanying the vicar over to his garden. Sure enough, there was Gertie sailing back and forth across the vicar's pond clearly enjoying getting into deep water. Not so me. After several abortive attempts to shoo her ashore I asked permission to wade in.

'Oh course, my dear sir. Do whatever you consider best to bring the current circumstances to a satisfactory conclusion,' sang the vicar who was stalking round the perimeter of the pond like a hungry heron. 'But I have to warn you, the construction of the pond is such that—'

It's too damn deep. Yes. The warning was too late. I'd already put one booted foot in and water had slurped over the top. Short of a miracle – like walking on the surface of the water which was wholly unlikely unless the reverend had powers of which I was unaware – I was not going to get within reach of Gertie. Revd Matthews had swayed to a halt and brought the palms of his hands together as if about to pray.

'It comes to me that I may have a solution to this current situation,' he said. 'They say "Lead us not into temptation" but there are certain circumstances where one may stray from the concept of the true meaning. Wait here.'

With his circumlocutory manner of speech I wondered how many parishioners Revd Matthews had managed to send off to sleep during his sermons as I watched him head down the garden, his trouser legs ballooning round his beanpole legs.

He returned clasping an armful of spinach leaves and began depositing little piles around the perimeter of the pond as if he were arranging prayer books. 'Perhaps these little offerings will be an inducement to our feathered friend to forsake the attractions of the open water for the more edible nature of these leaves.'

Gertie had stopped paddling and had her neck stretched over her back, her beak buried under one wing. Oh Lord, surely she hadn't dozed off, lulled into sleep by the vicar's words? But no. Her head reappeared. She'd only been preening. With a beady eye she watched the vicar finish his circle of leaves but remained bobbing in the middle of the pond.

In frustration I snatched up a leaf of spinach and waved it at her. 'Come on Gertie, move your—' I stopped myself just in time from doing an Eliza Dolittle at Ascot, aware the vicar was watching me. '...self,' I tailed off lamely.

But it did the trick. There was a sudden loud cackle from Gertie. With a powerful kick of her legs, she shot in full throttle towards me leaving a wake that slopped over the banks; springing out she showered me with water as she snatched the spinach from me.

'Well it seems my thoughts on the use of something of a vegetable nature have eventually borne the fruit of what we set out to do without too much effort,' said Revd Matthews.

'Yes. The spinach did the trick,' I agreed.

'You're going to have to do something about it,' said Lucy, when later we were discussing Gertie's wanderings over lunch. 'Otherwise we'll have the whole of Ashton up in arms. And it will be our goose that will well and truly be cooked.'

'Very funny,' I said, glaring at her. But of course she was right.

Eventually Gertie's forages to pastures new were curtailed by wiring, staking and tying an assortment of plastic mesh, chicken wire and dismantled budgerigar cages across the bottom of the garden to ensure all goose-sized holes were plugged. But it meant I had to sacrifice my newly established vegetable plot.

'Not to worry,' I said, putting on a brave face as I watched Gertie gobble up the last of my young lettuces and radishes. 'At least it's helping to fatten you up.'

Lucy winced. I knew she was getting rather fond of Gertie. She'd told me that every morning when she went down to let the goose out, there was a friendly honk. As the door to the potting shed was unlatched, Gertie would waddle out, eyes glinting; her head would immediately plunge into Lucy's pocket, rummaging for titbits. And she adored being tickled. With a honk of bliss, she would raise each wing in turn so that Lucy could scratch the soft down underneath.

As the summer slipped by, Lucy grew more and more concerned about Gertie's future. She tried hard to convince me that it would be better to opt for a turkey at Christmas.

'You do realize geese are very greasy,' she said. 'All that fat's not good for the digestion.'

'Lemon juice will soon fix that,' I said, not appreciating the depth of Lucy's feelings. Whoops.

Her eyes blazed as if an oak had erupted into a sea of green. There was an angry swish of her ponytail. Oh dear. I'd obviously said the wrong thing. 'You can cook the damn bird yourself then,' she said, storming out of the kitchen while I discretely closed the cordon bleu cookery book that I'd had open at 'Roast Goose à la Perigord'.

Matters weren't helped when one of the Stockwell sisters phoned up with a recipe for prune and apple stuffing that I had requested. Unfortunately Lucy took the call, and though she was polite enough to listen, all she scribbled on the telephone pad were a series of heavily inked-in daggers.

But I wasn't deterred. And Lucy began to realize that nothing was going to stop Gertie heading straight for the oven.

Mid-September, it was Mandy's twentieth birthday. She was going to head off down to her parents in Dorset for the weekend, but on the Friday, there was a little after-work celebration at Prospect House. Eric donated three bottles of wine and Beryl made a few sausage rolls and bought in some ready-made pizza slices. Crystal proposed a toast and we all drank to Mandy's health while she stood there, her face flushed with embarrassment. Having taken a few sips of wine, Crystal made her excuses and dragged Eric away just as he was about to refill his glass. There was an audible sigh of relief as we then set to and finished off the bottles between us.

It was gone ten by the time Lucy and I got back to Willow Wren. There were a couple of honks from the bottom of the garden as I fumbled with my keys in the dark, trying to sort out the front door Yale. When we finally managed to let ourselves in, we promptly tripped over Nelson, snoring in blissful deafness on the hall rug.

It had been a hectic day at the hospital, so Lucy was asleep as soon as her head hit the pillow. But I lay awake for what seemed like hours, tossing and turning. When I finally dozed off, I dreamt I was being chased round and round the kitchen by an irate goose with a knife and fork in each wing.

It was Gertie's honking that woke me up, the cackling rising to a crescendo.

'What the hell....' I spluttered, trying to shake off my drowsiness as I fumbled for my dressing-gown. Slinging it over my shoulders I pounded down the stairs, convinced that Foxie had Gertie by the throat.

An open back door greeted me, a pane of glass broken, the sound of footsteps running away. Too late, Nelson cottoned on to the fact that we'd had burglars and began to bark.

'Just think,' said Lucy brightly the following morning, 'if hadn't been for Gertie, heaven knows what they might have stolen.'

Though we hadn't much of value, I was a movie buff and did treasure my DVD collection. With that in mind I had to admit that Gertie had saved our skins; so the least we could do was save hers. So, yes. I now agreed with Lucy – it would be turkey for Christmas.

Gertie's future seemed even more secure when a couple of weeks later I was given two turkey poults to fatten up. Lucy found them quite endearing creatures. As they grew, so did her fondness for them.

'Besides,' she said, 'they're proving great company for Gertie.'

'I've been thinking,' she added as we watched the trio strut happily round the lawn. 'Perhaps we should just have boiled ham with all the trimmings for Christmas lunch.'

Fine, I thought, unless some client decided to give us a pig to fatten up. And if that became a pet as seemed likely, what then for Christmas lunch. Nut cutlets?

Chapter 7

The dry weather experienced during my first few weeks at Prospect House turned into a full-blown heatwave come August, which was good news for Westcott-on-Sea as it encouraged more trippers to travel the fifty miles or so down from London to take the sea air.

Not that sea air necessarily equated with fresh air. Though Westcott had the genteel trappings of a seaside resort – a little stuck in the fifties perhaps – with a pebbly beach, a wide promenade, small white-painted pier and pleasure gardens bedecked with scarlet geraniums – the pleasure to be gained from such attractions had to be balanced against the detractions of more unwelcome additions.

These took the form of piles of dark green bladderwrack washed up on the shore at this time of year; the swarms of black flies attracted to those piles,and the smell from them as they festered in the strong summer sun. It meant that the sea breezes gently blowing on shore, though cooling, were filled with the stench of rotting seaweed which, mixed with the smells from fish and chip shops, kebab and burger bars, drifted through the town causing many a visitor's brow to furrow, their noses to twitch, wondering if the public conveniences had become blocked. Prospect House was two miles inland but even that distance failed to prevent it from smelling like a fish market on an off day.

One Monday afternoon in particular was rank – not helped by my consulting-room window which I couldn't open due to layers of paint. So the window remained tightly shut. That, coupled with a waiting room full of fetid dog and cat breaths, not helped, I suspected, by one or two churning bowels, made for a rather rancid hour of consultations.

'I'm afraid your next appointment's not going to help matters,' said Beryl, holding up a can of 'Summer Bouquet' and spraying it vigorously over my head. I felt a mist of cloying cheap perfume descend on me making me smell like a walking lavatory block. 'It's a very excitable bull terrier. You'll need some help to hold her.'

Lucy was off-duty that afternoon.

'It means asking Mandy,' I said.

'So? It's part of her job,' said Beryl with a shrug. 'You're not afraid to ask her, are you?' she added, giving me one of her unblinking stares. Before I could reply she'd swivelled in her chair and called down the corridor. Mandy appeared out of the prep room. Beryl looked back at me, an eyebrow raised.

I cleared my throat. 'I'm wondering if you can give me a hand with the next patient,' I called out.

'Well, I'm busy getting the instruments ready for tomorrow. It's Crystal's ops morning,' Mandy replied, making no attempt to move.

Eric bustled into reception having just seen out his last appointment. 'Did I hear you say you needed some help, Paul?' he queried.

I nodded.

'Well Mandy can lend you a hand.' Eric beamed down the corridor at her. 'Can't you?'

'Of course, Eric. Just coming,' she replied.

Grrrrrr....

Beryl was right about the bull terrier. Blodwyn exuded heat the minute she pounded in, huffing and puffing, scrabbling and skittering. She was a prime example of her breed – built like a tank, well muscled, thick necked, with a broad egg-shaped head from which glinted deep-set, small button-black eyes. The only thing that spoilt her otherwise immaculate white coat were the numerous scars; you could almost tally them to her previous consultations for repairs to wounds ranging from those inflicted by neighbouring cats to a kick from a donkey over at an animal sanctuary in Chawcombe. Having made so many visits to the surgery, she was well known; her excitable temperament had been noted and underlined on her clinical records.

When Blodwyn steam-rollered in, Mandy and the dog's owner, Mrs Timms, came flying in with her. Mandy, her lips set in a sulky line, armpits stained dark green, was sent hurtling into the consulting table while Mrs Timms bounced off the door, lost a sandal and grabbed at my coat to save herself from plunging under the table. Blodwyn flung the full force of her weight against my shins and I boomeranged from Mrs Timms into Mandy's ample bosom. By the time we'd disentangled ourselves and wrestled Blodwyn onto the table, collapsing in a sweltering heap on top of her, the temperature felt as if it had soared several degrees.

'It's her ear,' gasped Mrs Timms, in between spitting out dog hairs. 'Blodwyn didn't see eye-to-eye with my cousin's Alsatian.'

While Mandy kept a vice-like grip on the dog's heaving bulk, I cautiously examined the jagged tear evident in Blodwyn's left ear.

'I'm afraid that will need stitching.' I said as Blodwyn swung round, her lolling tongue spraying me with spittle. 'Keep holding on,' I added, looking at a red-faced Mandy. 'You're doing a good job.' It didn't take a minute to draw up a shot of sedative, and it took just a few more for Blodwyn to become drowsy enough for us to manhandle her down to the prep room where she was given an intravenous injection and the torn ear stitched.

Just as I'd finished tying off the last suture, Beryl poked her head round the door, her hair like a layer of ravens' wings – all of a flap. 'Paul,' she said in a loud whisper, hand to the side of her face, 'would you be able to see a fish for me?'

I felt like saying 'Only if it's small fry' but the look on Beryl's pinched face suggested I'd be wise not to bait her. I merely shrugged which she took as my acceptance. With another quick squirt of 'Summer Bouquet' aimed in my direction she disappeared back up to reception.

I could have tried 'It all sounds a bit fishy to me' on Mandy, but she was in no mood for jokes and the shark-eyed look she gave me warned me off.

But it was no joke when, half-an-hour later, the golden orf landed on my consulting table in a large plastic bucket. To my inexperienced eye, it looked like a giant goldfish with dull orange scales, speckled black, and drooping tail and fins, spotted red. It hung motionless in the water, a large gash clearly visible near the base of its tail. Mr Chang, its owner, was a lithe young man who, I understood from Beryl, ran the Kowloon Curry House in the centre of Westcott.

'You never know,' she'd said. 'If you sort his fish out he might let you have a Chinese on the house.'

Mr Chang was olive-skinned, with narrow hooded eyes and jet-black hair that stuck up like hedgehog spikes. He extracted a paper napkin edged with red and yellow dragons from his jeans and mopped his face.

'Velly hot,' he said.

I agreed.

'And velly smelly.' His broad, snub nose twitched.

I nodded again. 'And the fish?'

'Velly sick. We have large tank in window. Velly big.' To empha-size the point, Mr Chang stretched out his arms. 'Car crash into window. Break glass like so.' He raised his hand and brought it swiftly down on the table in a karate chop. Water slopped out of the bucket. 'All fish velly frightened. This fish sliced.'

Sliced? Filleted? Battered? I had a brief mental image of orf and chips before realizing an 'Ah so....' had escaped from my lips. I quickly covered my slip of the tongue by saying: 'Ah ... so the fish got cut by a shard of glass.'

Mr Chang's dark eyes stared intently at me. 'You put light?'

'I'll do my best,' I said, completely in the dark. How on earth did you stitch up a fish?

Beryl watched, her one eye agog, as I struggled down to the prep room with the heavy bucket. Sliding it onto the table, I stepped back and bit my lip. Now what? I peered down at the fish as it slowly circled round and round.

Mandy bobbed through. She must have seen me rubbing my chin. 'You going to anaesthetize it then?' she said.

'Er ... well ...yes....'

'Crystal uses Alka-Seltzers.'

'Oh she does, does she?'

'I've got some up in the flat if you want.'

'Please.'

When she returned, I took the tube from her, unscrewed the cap and tipped three tablets into my palm.

'Crystal would use four in a bucket that size,' said Mandy.

I tipped out another tablet.

'Probably five, thinking about it,' said Mandy.

Without comment, I tipped out a fifth and tossed the handful into the bucket.

Within seconds, it was a sea of bubbles. The fizzing continued unabated, the surface of the water a white cauldron with no way of seeing what effect it was having on the fish. Twenty minutes later the water had calmed down. So had the orf. Having succumbed to the initial explosion of carbon dioxide, it was very calm. Too calm to my mind. On its side, gills scarcely moving, it looked half-dead. Whatever, I had to fish it out. Rolling up my sleeves, I immersed my arms in to the gently fizzing water and cupped my hands under the orf's belly, gradually raising it to the surface. But as soon as the surface of the water was broken, the fish slipped out of my fingers and flopped back in with a splash.

Mandy held up a square of muslin.

'Crystal always uses this,' she said in a casual manner, as if it was the most obvious thing to think of. So why hadn't I thought of it?

I snatched the material from her and pushed it into the bucket and under the fish. I have to confess it did make it much easier. With the orf netted, I was able to drag it out and carry it through to the oper-ating theatre where I plopped it on the table, rivulets of water running across to drip onto the floor.

Mandy now held up a wet green drape. 'Crystal always wraps this round the fish. Stops it drying out.'

'Right!' I plucked the drape from her and folded it round the orf just leaving the damaged flank exposed. The wound was deeper than I'd suspected, extending from behind the tail to within a few inches of the dorsal fin. Now what? I saw Mandy open her mouth. 'Crystal always uses....' I expected her to say. But she didn't say a word; merely opened an emergency pack of instruments from which I extracted a sterile drape, spread it on the trolley and allowed her to tip the pack out.

Despite having the Venetian blinds closed to the glare and heat of the sun, the theatre was hot and I knew I'd have to work quickly before the fish dried out. I threaded a needle and jabbed it into one side of the wound. The needle bounced off the skin. I tried again. The same thing happened.

'Needle must be blunt,' I declared, throwing it to one side.

I threaded another one. That needle buckled and snapped in half as I tried forcing it through the fish's flesh. 'What's wrong with these bloody needles?' I said, feeling myself getting hot under the collar, a trickle of sweat running down my back. Though the fish wasn't in a flap I certainly was.

Mandy glowered at me, her cheeks a deeper shade of scarlet. 'It's not the needles,' she said.

'Really?' My tone was sarcastic.

'No. Fish have got tough skin. Crystal always uses one of those.' She pointed to the largest needle at the end of the row. To my mind it was more suitable for suturing a Great Dane than a fish but I wasn't going to carp on about it. If Mandy said....

I still had trouble pulling the wound together. Flakes of flesh kept breaking off, each one accompanied by a tut from the ever-watchful Mandy. The suture material snapped a couple of times provoking more tuts. I began to feel more like a fish out of water than the wretched fish in front of me. The word 'flounder' sprang to mind several times. However, I eventually managed to draw the edges of the wound together; and once sewn up, the orf was slid back into a bucket of fresh water.

'Make sure it's at room temperature,' Mandy said.

Yes, Mandy, yes, I thought. Otherwise both me and the fish will end up in hot water. How orf-ful. Yes … well. I jabbed my finger in the bucket. Testing times … testing times....

Now I had to wait while the fish swam back into consciousness. Only it didn't appear to want to. It remained motionless, floating just under the surface of the water. No sign of life. Not a flicker of tail or fin. Nothing. A bubble of panic rose in my throat. Perhaps the fish had been out of the water too long? Maybe all my poking and prodding had been too much for it?

Mandy hovered into view. Here we go again, I thought. Mandy says. 'Yes? What is it?' I snapped.

Mandy pursed her lips and then said, 'Crystal always bubbles some oxygen through afterwards.'

I was dying to say 'Well, Paul says "No", but realized that would be counterproductive. Mandy was baiting me but I wasn't going to be hooked. 'Fetch the machine in then.'

With a smug smile, she marched out and returned, wheeling the anaesthetic trolley behind her. She unhooked the tubing from the oxygen cylinder and immersed the end of it in the bucket, turning on the valve as she did so. Gas immediately began to bubble through the water. With one hand, Mandy moved the tube to direct the gas flow over the fish's mouth and gills while with the other, she grasped the fish's tail and propelled it backwards and forwards. Clearly she knew what she was doing. Within minutes, the orf flicked its tail and shot out of Mandy's hand, thumped into the side of the bucket and then began to swim round it.

Mr Chang was delighted with the outcome. 'Thank you velly velly much,' he sang. 'Please come to my restaurant. Meal on me.'

When he'd gone, Beryl said, 'That will be something to look forward to. I gather they do a very good spread there. Set price for as much as you can eat on Sundays,' she added, as she accompanied me down to the office on her way out for a quick ciggie. 'King prawns, chop suey, foo yung. The full works.' She patted her stomach. 'I guess you'd have to have a strong digestive system to make the most of it.'

'And if you didn't, then these could come in handy.' Mandy had appeared at the doorway, holding up the tube of Alka-Seltzers. 'They'd soon settle you down.' She rattled the tube at me.

Hmm. It would take more than just tablets, my girl, to settle me down. Much more. I was beginning to appreciate how Lucy felt.

The hot weather continued with no respite. Equally, there was no respite from Blodwyn. Two days after having had her left ear stitched, she was back with a nick in her right one. Lucy was on hand to help control the bull terrier this time: Mandy made sure of that.

'Had a bit of a set-too with a chihuahua just down the road from here,' said Mrs Timms, as Lucy locked limbs with Blodwyn on the table.

'A chihuahua? The owner didn't happen to be a lady with platinum blonde hair?' I asked.

'Why yes ... Mrs Paget. Do you know her?'

'Had digs with her for a while.'

'Paul....' Lucy gave me a pleading look as Blodwyn buckled beneath her.

'Oh you must be the young man she rather fancied.' Mrs Timms suddenly stopped and went bright red. 'Chico's fine,' she went on, rapidly changing the subject. 'It's just Blodwyn.'

'Paul.' Lucy's voice had taken on a more threatening tone.

I quickly turned my attention to the dog.

The tear in the ear was relatively minor. I could have stitched it but wasn't keen to subject Blodwyn to another anaesthetic so soon after the last one. I explained this to Mrs Timms and we agreed to leave the wound to repair of its own accord. Now both of Blodwyn's ears drooped.

'At least they match,' exclaimed Mrs Timms, before she was whisked out of the door. She was whisked back before the end of the week.

'It's his eye this time,' shouted Mrs Timms, above a boisterous bark from Blodwyn. I gripped the consulting table to prevent myself from crashing to the floor as Blodwyn careered into me. 'When I let her out last thing there was this terrible commotion. I think our neighbour's cat must have strayed into the garden.'

'It should have had more sense,' I muttered, as in a sea of flying fur Blodwyn was levered onto the table. On this occasion both Mandy and Lucy were co-opted to lend a hand. Even so, it was still a struggle with Blodwyn squirming around beneath them. I nervously peered at her partially closed left eye.

'Did the cat get him?' asked Mrs Timms.

'Looks like it.' I gently pressed on the lower lid to evert the conjunctiva. It was red and swollen. Something protruded. I fetched a pair of artery forceps and holding them up in front of the dog's face said, 'Everyone ready?'

'I guess so,' replied Lucy, her voice muffled in the hair of Blodwyn's back. Mandy had one arm under the dog's chin, forcing her head against her while her free hand was constantly fighting to control the front paws which were skimming to and fro across the table. 'Ready as I'll ever be,' she spluttered.

I cautiously pulled down the lower lid again, opened the teeth of the forceps and fastened them on the foreign body I'd spotted lodged in the conjunctiva. Blodwyn howled. She swung away. Lucy, Mandy and Mrs Timms were dragged across the room in a screech of table legs while I was left holding the evidence. The tip of a cat's claw.

With still no sign of the heatwave diminishing, another hot, sticky meeting with Blodwyn loomed.

Beryl was apologetic. 'Sorry, Paul, 'she said. 'It's a house visit this time. Mrs Timms just can't get her in.'

As I stood waiting for Mrs Timms to answer her door, the sun ferociously beat down. Rivulets of sweat ran between my shoulder blades. I shivered despite the heat, not relishing the thought of trying to handle Blodwyn on my own.

'We were up on the Downs,' said Mrs Timms, ushering me into the lounge. 'Blodwyn spotted a pheasant and gave chase into the bracken. Now she can hardly stand.' She stood in front of the fireplace, her hands clicking through the row of pearls round her neck.

This time there was no boisterous greeting from Blodwyn; no shaking of the massive head; no lolling of the tongue: nothing. She was lying stretched out on the hearth rug, panting heavily, her body quivering. There was only the merest flick of her tail as I bent down to examine her.

'When did all this happen?'

'About an hour ago. I heard this yelp and she came rushing back to me. By the time we'd got home she'd collapsed.' Mrs Timms knelt down and cradled the dog's head. But it wasn't necessary. Blodwyn had no interest in what was going on. All her zest, her bounce, had vanished. Clearly something was drastically wrong. But what?

I ran my hand down her back and noticed her left hind leg appeared swollen.

'Help me roll her over,' I instructed. With Blodwyn levered onto her side and her right leg pushed back, I was able to examine the inside of her left thigh where with less hair, the mottled red and purple bruising was more obvious – as were the two minute puncture wounds.

'She's been bitten by an adder,' I exclaimed, jumping to my feet. 'That explains her state of shock.' I opened my black bag. 'But don't worry, we'll get her sorted out.' I gave Blodwyn an anti-inflammatory injection and promised to visit again the next day.

It was another scorcher.

'Well, how is she?' I enquired, standing in the lounge, my shirt wet and sticking to my back – the result of nerves more than the heat. There was no sign of Blodwyn.

Mrs Timms was about to reply when I heard a pounding on the patio. A familiar skittering of nails. A familiar huffing and puffing. I scarcely had time to turn around before thirty kilos of well-muscled bull terrier tore through the French windows and rammed into the back of my legs. I was sent spinning onto the carpet. Tongue lolling, tail wagging furiously, Blodwyn stood over me and gave a deep bay of excitement.

'Well … well….' said Mrs Timms, with a nervous little laugh. 'She's obviously bowled over to see you.'

Still flattened on the carpet, all I could do was grunt – too stumped for a reply.

Chapter 8

The spell of hot weather finally broke; and with it the stench of seaweed was washed away by a series of heavy thunderstorms. Instead of hot, panting pooches coming through the surgery, I was subjected to wet, mud-splattered mutts that shook their coats, showering mine in brown spots, before sitting to the commands of their dishevelled owners, both pets and owners quietly steaming.

Indirectly, through those thunderstorms, another creature turned up to disrupt my daily routine.

In the top corner of the Green, just opposite Prospect House, stood an oak tree – just the one solitary specimen and not the best example of its type. The spread of its boughs was far from the one conjured up by royal oaks depicted in the spread of glossy *Country Living* magazines. No majestic canopy for this oak – that was never going to happen, as over the years various branches that were deemed a threat to the road alongside had been unceremoniously chopped off, leaving the tree with a decidedly lopsided look. Nevertheless it was old and had clung on despite the fact it was now surrounded by the suburban sprawl of Westcott. And I certainly enjoyed my glimpses of it from the operating theatre – in the odd moment or two snatched between spays and dentals.

So I was quite sympathetic when Beryl appeared one coffee break waving a piece of paper at me rather than the tail end of her mid-morning cigarette.

'You'll sign, won't you, Paul?' she said, thrusting the paper at me. 'It's a petition to save the oak tree on the Green. After all, it's part of Westcott's heritage. It needs to be protected.' She gave me a one-eyed glare and pushed a pen under my nose.

As I added my signature to the long list I noticed several familiar names including those of Cynthia Paget and the Adamses from over at the Woolpack. My, my, Beryl had certainly been busy. Didn't realize such passion lurked under that thick crust of make-up.

'To think, it's been here all these hundreds of years,' Beryl was saying. 'Cynthia reckons Elizabeth 1st could have ridden under it. Had a tryst or two with her Earl of Leicester.'

That, I thought, was stretching credulity. Cynthia must have been reading too many historical romances. Even if good Queen Bess had chosen to visit this area – and several manors in West Sussex laid claim to her having slept at least one night in those houses – Westcott in her day would have been non-existent, just sheep pasture with a few tracts of woodland. Besides which, the oak would have been just a sapling – more likely to be ridden over than under. Still, I didn't want to dent any romantic illusions so I nodded in agreement.

'And, of course, the local dogs love it,' I said, thinking in more practical terms. I knew it was the daily highlight of Mrs Paget's outing – or rather that of her chihuahua, Chico. He always made a beeline for the tree, saving his full bladder until he could cock his leg as high up the tree's bole as he could lift it. No doubt while she daydreamed of a tryst with Dudley.

'What's this about dogs?' It was Eric. He'd bounded in, somewhat breathless.

'We were talking about the oak on the Green,' said Beryl.

'Oh that old thing. Absolute menace. Should have been chopped down yonks ago.'

I saw Beryl's eye contract, her lips followed suit; she was clearly squaring up for battle. 'Er ... Eric....' I said, in an attempt to forestall a confrontation, but Eric had got the wind behind him and was in full sail.

He looked from Beryl to me. 'In fact, that's why I'm late. There's some nutters from the local history society parading around out there with banners, blocking the road, causing a traffic jam. Absolute waste of time if you ask me.'

'I was about to,' said Beryl, the tone of her voice decidedly cutting – it could have felled the oak in one stroke.

Oh Lord, I thought. If the tree wasn't going for the chop, Eric certainly was.

'You were?' said Eric, still unaware of his impending toppling. 'So what's this all about?' He took the sheet of paper Beryl had been waving at him and was just about to read it when Crystal appeared.

My Julie Andrews, as always, smart, bubbly, breezing in on a cloud of delicate perfume.

She intervened. 'It's Beryl's petition to save the oak. I've already signed. Must do our bit, Eric.'

'We certainly must, mustn't we?' Beryl was jabbing the biro at Eric like a rapier in a duel. 'So you'll sign?'

'Of course, he will,' said Crystal, flashing her a smile.

Of course, he will, I thought.

'Of course, I will,' said Eric, snatching up the pen with a grunt and dashing off his signature – an illegible scrawl.

'And print your name next to it,' said Beryl, head on one side, watching him like a hawk – a one-eyed one.

He duly obliged.

In the event he needn't have bothered. In the last of the thunderstorms of that week, the oak was struck by lightning; it split in two, with one half collapsing onto the Green, the other leaning precariously over the road. There was no question of its preservation other than as firewood. The council were in like a bevy of beavers, the whine of their chainsaws echoing through Prospect House all morning. As the tree went out of our life so the baby squirrel came into it.

Two young lads, wearing baseball caps and Harry Potter T-shirts brought him in. He'd been rescued from the hollow bole of the oak as the last of it was felled.

I carefully opened the shoe-box they'd slid onto the consulting table, parted the cotton wool and stared down at the vivid pink-skinned creature barely two inches long curled up inside. The most conspicuous features were the dark bulges of unopened eyes and huge claw-like feet.

'It was in a large sort of nest,' chirruped one of the boys, standing on tiptoe to peer into the box.

'But we don't think it was a bird's nest,' said the other lad, leaning over his friend's shoulder. 'And it doesn't look like a bird.'

'Of course it's not a bird,' hissed his mate, squirming round. 'It's got four legs. Birds have only got two.'

'I know that. I'm not daft.'

'So it's not a bird.'

'Didn't say it was.'

'It's a baby squirrel,' I said, hastily intervening.

'There. Told you it wasn't a bird,' said the shorter of the boys, looking up at his friend.

'But you didn't know what it was,' he retorted.

'Nor did you.'

'Didn't say I did. I just knew it wasn't a bird.'

'Anyone could have worked that out, dick-head.'

'Now, now boys. Let's decide what we do with the squirrel, shall we?' I tapped the side of the box. The boys fell silent and stared up at me from beneath the brims of their caps.

'Would either of you be able to look after him?'

Both shook their heads. Uhmm. I was afraid this was going to happen. But no doubt Beryl could track down a local animal rescue centre with the expertise to rear a baby squirrel. But I hadn't reckoned on Lucy.

'Ah, isn't he sweet?' she declared, as soon as she set eyes on him. All talk of rescue centres was dismissed as she set about constructing an artificial drey from an empty drugs carton with an infra-red lamp suspended above it.

'Cyril needs two-hourly feeding to start with,' she informed me.'

'Cyril?'

'Cyril – squirrel. Why not?'

Hmm. It would be Ducky Lucky and Turkey Lurky next if we weren't too careful. Though I wouldn't mind a juicy Lucy.

'Paul?'

'Sorry. Just thinking…. What are you going to feed him on?'

'Milkocat,' said Lucy, her voice full of confidence. She brandished a tin of milk powder in front of me.

'That's for rearing kittens,' I said, a tad too smugly.

She glowered at me. 'I'm well aware of that. But I'm sure it will do the trick.'

I was far from convinced. 'And how do you propose to get the stuff into him? It's not going to be easy.' God. I was beginning to sound like a real Jonah.

'With this,' she said, waving a pipette at me.

I was about to tell her that she'd find it difficult, but decided I'd said enough already. Let her find out for herself.

She did. 'Blast.' She swore as milk shot across the squirrel's mouth and squirted out the other side.

'I know what you're thinking,' she said, looking daggers at me.

I held up my hands.

'Didn't say a word.'

'Didn't have to.'

I don't think she really knew what I was thinking. My little juicy Lucy.

I stepped back as Mandy marched into the prep room with the usual snap and crackle of her starched uniform.

'What's all this?' she said. 'Not falling out are we? All because of a baby squirrel. Can't have that.' Her face was a picture of innocence.

Liar. I knew damn'd well she'd love to see us scrapping.

'It's nothing we can't sort out,' said Lucy.

Mandy smiled sweetly. What saccharine smugness. Pure Mandy-candy. 'Let's try a syringe shall we?'

That didn't work either. More milk seemed to spray over the squirrel's eyes, nose and body than actually went down his throat.

'You're not holding him properly,' declared Mandy, after several abortive attempts.

'Well, if you think you can do better, you hold him,' retorted Lucy.

Uh ... uh.... there was that tension again – that antagonism bubbling up between them.

Better to be out of all this I thought and quietly tiptoed out.

'We need a teat to suckle,' Lucy told me when morning surgery was finished.

Mmm. Yes, my juicy Lucy. I'd love to have a suckle.

'Paul! Why are you leering at me?'

'Sorry. Nothing. Just thinking you won't find one small enough,' I said. I got the 'Lucy look' for my efforts. Her stubborn, don't-stand-in-my-way look.

She returned after a lunchtime trip into Westcott, her mood buoyant, her voice distinctly triumphant. 'This is the answer.' She waved a baby doll's feeding set at me.

I remained unconvinced until I saw the baby rodent, curled up fast asleep, his stomach full, bulging out like a white balloon. Full marks to Lucy then. But she hadn't finished.

'You know that cat down in the ward. The one that's just had kittens.'

'Er ... yes.'

'She's boarding for a while, isn't she?'

'You'd need to check with Beryl, but I think she's in for a couple of weeks. Why?'

'Oh, it's just something I've been reading up on.' Lucy tapped the open book she'd borrowed from the hospital library as she sat drinking her afternoon mug of tea. 'Says here how an orphaned squirrel was fostered onto a cat with kittens.'

'Lucy, I don't somehow think....'

That look came into her eyes again. Useless for me to say more.

With Cyril lined up alongside the three kittens lying next to their mother, I unwisely expressed my doubts again. This wasn't going to work. The cat would surely snap at the baby squirrel and pull it away. 'Shh,' was all I got from Lucy as we watched the mother give her kittens a protective lick. She then sniffed the squirrel. Lucy's hand hovered just inches away, ready to snatch Cyril up in case he was attacked. There was another tentative sniff. Then another as the cat's head lowered towards the wriggling pink body.

'Lucy....'

'Shh.'

Suddenly the cat's tongue darted out; the naked squirrel was lightly touched and then fervently licked as the cat started washing him. Lick. Lick. Lick. Back and forth went the tongue over the tiny, pink body, transferring scent. Cyril had been accepted.

Now there was the question of getting Cyril to suckle. Cats' nipples are large. A squirrel's mouth small, the jaws quite rigid and with two large pointed bottom incisors already well developed. This was going to be no easy task. But then Lucy still had that look so....

He was suckling twenty minutes later.

Within three days his eyes opened.

'You'll really have to watch him now,' I warned.

Cyril scrabbled up the side of the cat basket using his large claws to grip. Once on top, he tottered along, rolling from side to side like a drunken sailor, his tail trailing behind him.

This task became easier as he grew stronger. You'd see him scuttling along the top of the basket, his tail now curled over his back, his gait less rolling now that he'd gained strength in his muscles. Soon he was moving like an adult squirrel: wild, erratic; a sudden stop; a dash in another direction.

One morning as I was doing my ward round, Lucy let the mother cat out of her kennel to allow her to stretch her legs. Cyril also slipped out and zig-zagged up and down the corridor. I guess something in his jerky movements triggered an instinctive reaction in the cat. For I suddenly saw her tense, crouch, eyes wide open, ears flat against her head, the tip of her tail twitching. There was no doubt as to her intentions. She was about to pounce. And Cyril was going to be her victim. He, oblivious to his impending demise, had stopped to have a good scratch. Then he was off again. Darting down the ward. All too much for the cat. She leapt into the air, claws outstretched.

'Lucy,' I cried.

She was at the sink, washing bowls, her back to the unfolding drama. At my shout, she spun round, just as the cat sailed past her. With a loud crash, the bowl she was holding dropped from her soapy hands to the floor. It startled the cat sufficient for her to misjudge her leap. She skidded past Cyril. Lucy pounced, throwing herself on the cat and skilfully pinning her down, while the bowl spun down the corridor, ringing against the metal doors of the kennels.

Cyril skittered through the bars of a kennel housing a bewildered Westie who immediately started yapping, joined in seconds later by the howls and yowls of several other startled dogs.

Into this cacophony walked Crystal. She stood, hands on hips, at the end of the corridor. Her voice sliced through the air. 'What on earth is going on down here?'

It was if someone had flicked a switch. The barking died away immediately. The Westie gave two additional, hesitant woofs and then he too fell silent with a nervous gulp.

Crystal clipped down the corridor until level with me. 'Well, Paul? Perhaps you can explain.' She stared at me intently.

Oh those eyes of hers. Those cornflower-blue eyes. Such beautiful eyes. Such … well, actually they now looked rather thunderous, the sort of blue seen in clouds about to hit you between the eyes with a heavy burst of hail.

'Er … well, it was the squirrel,' I responded in a hoarse whisper, pointing down at Cyril who'd come hopping up to Crystal's ankles.

Oh what lovely ankles. So finely turned. Such delicate feet. Pink lacquered toes peeping from sandals like blushing maids all in a row. More like a string of nuts to judge from the keen interest Cyril was taking in them. And nuts were for eating. Oh no. Those razor-sharp teeth of his.

Crystal looked down and took a genteel step to the side. Phew.

'Oh, yes. This squirrel. Time it was found a home, don't you think? We don't want it taking up unnecessary space. Or too much of our staff's time.'

So there we had it – Crystal clear.

Time for Cyril to move on. I had to admit there was no excuse for him staying as he was now eating and drinking of his own accord. But where was he to go?

I had a sneaking feeling a decision had already been made. That look on Lucy's face said it all. When I hesitantly suggested one or two rescue centres based in West Sussex or Westcott's Wildlife Park, the look intensified.

'But we're stuffed to overflowing,' I said, as the words 'Willow Wren' were finally voiced by Lucy. 'Where could we put him?'

'He could go in with the two pheasants and one-legged crow.'

'The mesh isn't rodent-proof.'

'You could soon fix that.'

'Me?'

'You.' She gave me her 'Lucy look'.

I fixed the mesh the next day and Cyril moved in the day after.

He was greeted with a few squawks from the pheasants; and the crow gave him a funny Beryl-like stare. But ruffled feathers were soon smoothed and the quartet settled down to a summer together.

Cyril became quite addicted to the pelleted chicken feed on offer. And he certainly became very tame.

'Sweet, isn't he?' said Lucy, standing in the aviary with Cyril on her shoulder.

In his paws, he was turning over his favourite titbit – a custard cream – busily gnawing away at it, his cheeks rapidly filling with biscuit.

And he was soon able to fend for himself. The skill with which he demonstrated his ability to construct a drey was proof of that. Another of Lucy's looks made sure I knocked up a nest box for him. She provided the straw.

Now Cyril was in his element, racing down to yank up a pile of stems in his mouth, scuttling back up to the box where he'd sit chewing them up, weaving them into a nest. He'd bury himself in it, just his head poking out of the matted straw, his teeth clacking like a sewing-machine should you go too near.

'So, are you going to let him go?' asked Beryl.

'You're not going to keep him, surely?' asked Mandy.

Even Eric tossed in a question in passing.

Crystal's pink, Cupid-bow lips remained sealed.

Here was a dilemma. Cyril was self-sufficient and I felt sure he'd like a mate. Yet grey squirrels are very destructive and it hardly seemed fair to release him in nearby woods where he could do enormous damage to young trees and possibly be shot in the process. It was Cyril himself who provided the answer.

Lucy came running indoors to where I was stretched out on the sofa trying to tackle the crossword in the paper.

With a gulp she said, 'It's Cyril. Can't find him anywhere. He must have escaped. Come on. We must go and look for him.'

Well, yes. I suppose we should, I thought. On the other hand, perhaps it was a blessing in disguise that he'd made off. Saved us the problem of deciding what to do with him.

Lucy interrupted my musings. 'You just going to laze there all day, or what?' She dashed through to the kitchen saying she was getting some custard creams.

There followed an excruciating half an hour which saw the two of us trailing round the perimeter of Ashton's recreation ground, gazing up into the branches of the sycamores, poking through overgrown clumps of leylandii calling out 'Cyril' while our outstretched hands each held a custard cream.

'This is ridiculous,' I exclaimed to Lucy, as yet another passer-by, having asked what we were looking for, gave us a look of pity as we told him 'Cyril the squirrel' and walked on no doubt thinking we'd been reading too much Beatrix Potter. And when a youth in knee-holed jeans rode by on his bike with a snigger and I overhead him on the corner telling his mates of us two nutters on the rec. I decided enough was enough and called a halt to the search.

Lucy did one final 'Coo ... eee' in the direction of the ash tree that fronted the rectory and waved a custard cream at Revd Matthews when he hoved into view. He gave a hesitant wave back.

A week later, I was taking Nelson for a totter across the rec., his arthritic limbs only capable of carrying him once round the perimeter. One of Ashton's senior citizens who'd also been out for a totter, was now sitting on the one bench that had yet to be vandalized. Despite it only being early October and the weather still balmy, she was wrapped in a camel-coloured coat several sizes too big for her which made her look like a sack of potatoes. To her side was a white, plastic bag sporting the name of a well-known supermarket. Behind her, running up and down the back of the bench were three squirrels. All Cyril look-a-likes. As I stopped to watch, she extracted an endless stream of food from the bag. Lumps of cheese. Broken wafers. Biscuits. The squirrels scuttled back and forth reaching down to snatch each item offered without the slightest trace of fear.

'Such pretty creatures, aren't they?' she said, peering up at me from the depths of her sack.

I nodded, yanking Nelson back as he pulled forward in an attempt to hoover up the crumbs.

'And so tame,' she added. 'Especially this dear little chap.' She glanced down at the squirrel who'd jumped onto her arm and was now clasping the biscuit she'd given him.

Though he looked like the other two, bright-eyed, bushy-tailed, tubby little tummy – all the attributes of a healthy squirrel – there was something about him which made me think he could be Cyril. For a moment I couldn't decide what that something was. Then it came to me. It was the way he was devouring the biscuit held in his paws. How those incisors were crunching through it. The way it was rapidly disappearing into his mouth. No other squirrel could surely enjoy a biscuit with such relish as he did.

Yes, it had to be Cyril.

And what clinched it?

Why, the biscuit being eaten: a custard cream of course.

Chapter 9

I was a mite suspicious when one late July morning, just before the start of the day's appointments, I saw Eric hovering at the end of the corridor outside my consulting-room.

'Ah Paul. Just the man,' he cried, with a flourish of his arms. The joviality in his voice did nothing to allay my doubts. Eric was an amiable enough fellow but usually only became civil around coffee-break time. This was far too early for him. Something was up.

'Before you start, I'd like a word,' he went on, pointing a finger through the door. 'Just the two of us.' He disappeared into the room. By the time I'd got there several scenarios had galloped through my brain. I remembered the tête-à-tête I'd had with Crystal just before they'd both bombed off to Venice leaving me with the Richardsons' horse. Was I about to be forewarned about some particular client of Eric's? The Stockwells for instance. According to Beryl, they would have no one but him. There again, perhaps I'd upset someone. Put my foot in it. No. Surely not. Eric seemed more adept at doing that than me. Besides it would be Crystal wagging the admonishing finger. Not Eric. Puzzled I entered the room.

'Close the door,' said Eric. 'This won't take a moment.' He was standing by the examination table, shirt ballooning over his belt which had slipped down over his paunch so that his trousers had dropped, the crotch now nearly at knee level. I'd often compared Eric to a ball, the way he bounced around the place, throwing himself into his work with boundless energy, but today, with the sagging clothes, he looked more reminiscent of a half-deflated one discarded on the beach, the image of which a blue, red and yellow striped tie loose round his neck, did nothing to dispel.

He cleared his throat while reaching across to the instrument trolley where he picked up a thermometer and rolled it between his fingers. 'I'm not quite sure how to put this,' he went on.

I gave a surreptitious glance at my watch. There were only minutes to go before surgery started and already I could hear a dog yapping in reception. Soon it would be Beryl snapping at me, wondering where I'd got to. Hurry up, Eric. Say what you have to say.

He dropped the thermometer on the trolley and turned back to me. 'I was playing golf yesterday afternoon with Alex Ryman. He's one of our clients.'

Yes. Yes. And? There was a cat now miaowing in the waiting-room.

'We sort of had a set-too at the fourth green. About one of his putts. I won't go into the details.'

Better not, Eric. Otherwise the waiting-room will be overflowing.

'Well, anyway, I don't somehow think I'd be welcome if a vet's needed over at his smallholding in the next few days.'

'Is that likely?' I asked.

'It's a possibility.'

Here we go. What's about to foal, whelp, litter or calf down I wonder?

'It's the Rymans' pig.'

'Pig?'

'Their saddleback. It's due to farrow soon. Not that there should be any problem. But you never know.'

'Er ... couldn't Crystal....?' I faltered.

The look of horror that flashed up on Eric's face said it all. Pigs, it seemed, weren't her cup of tea. Something she preferred to leave to him. Or, as of now, to me – until such time Alex Ryman and Eric were back on par – golf buddies once more. Mmm.

'How soon's soon?' I asked.

'Alex reckons in the next forty-eight hours or so. But he might be wrong.' Eric gave an embarrassed little harrumph. 'So you don't mind covering this one for me?'

Seems I had no choice, especially when he went on to tell me he'd already forewarned Beryl. 'She's keeping it under wraps. I'd rather Crystal didn't find out. Could be a bit awkward. You know how it is.'

Uh. So not only was I liable to see this pig of Eric's I was also having to save his bacon. Oh well, such was an assistant's life.

*

Just after lunch the following day, I breezed into reception to be greeted by a loud 'Psst' from Beryl and a beckoning from an uncompromising vermilion nail.

'Here,' she whispered, hunched furtively behind the computer screen.

I stepped across to the reception desk as her glass eye swivelled up to the ceiling while her good one glanced anxiously round the empty room. 'It's on,' she said.

'What?'

She hissed, 'You know.' She held a hand up to the right side of her mouth. The words came out muffled. 'Operation porker.'

'You mean....'

'Shh ... yes. I've booked you in a visit. Two-thirty.'

'So how's the afternoon shaping up?' It was Crystal.

Both Beryl and I started and sprang apart as she approached the desk.

'Fine ... fine,' stuttered Beryl, her fingers skimming over the keyboard, the Rymans' case history sliding quickly off the screen. 'You've got Mrs Frobisher – the Lord Mayor's wife – at three. Her two Swedish elkhounds are due for their boosters.'

And I've got a pig due for farrowing I thought glumly.

Before I left for the Rymans, Beryl sneaked down to the office and slipped a folded scrap of paper into my hand. 'Directions of how to get there,' she whispered before tiptoeing out. She was clearly enjoying this little bit of subterfuge and I wondered whether she expected me to memorize the directions and then swallow the ball of paper.

As it turned out, I was thankful for those directions. The Rymans' smallholding was in the next village along from Ashton, one called Chawcombe. It wasn't so much a village as a straggle of houses along a busy road that ran parallel to the north side of the Downs and from which numerous lanes ran off in to the countryside. I'd have run off several had it not been for Beryl's red inked map with Natt's Lane clearly marked and an asterisk next to Downside Cottage – a bit of a misnomer as I discovered, since the cottage was several miles away from the Downs and wasn't a cottage but a bungalow. One from the 1950s, built of plain red brick with concrete roof tiles to which a 1970s' flat-roofed loft extension had been added, hung-tiled in a mismatch of dark brown. As I drove into the tarmac drive and rounded the corner of the bungalow I half-expected to see a conservatory. And yes, there it was. A white PVC bubble of glass stuck to the back like a blob of used chewing gum, and from it strode a woman, followed closely by a boy of about eight and a girl who looked a year or so younger.

'Jill Ryman,' she said, introducing herself with the shake of a hand. She was tall, in her mid-thirties, thin as fuse wire, breasts flat as paper, wearing grubby overalls and wellington boots. 'And this is Emily and Joshua. Say hello to Mr....?'

'Paul Mitchell.'

Emily looked up at me through metal-rimmed glasses and smiled shyly exposing two missing front teeth, but it was Joshua who spoke. 'Miss Piggy's having babies.' He studied me through a mop of tousled brown hair, his dark eyes unflinching.

'Yes. Well, so I understand,' I said, somewhat unnerved by the intensity of the lad's expression. I lifted out my black bag. 'Let's hope she doesn't need too much help.'

Emily suddenly found her voice. 'Is that for the babies?' she lisped, pointing.

'Well, yes, I suppose it is,' I replied with a chuckle, conjuring up a picture of a bag stuffed full of piglets.

She giggled. Joshua remained silent, his lips curled down – clearly it was no laughing matter for this young man.

'Now, Emily, don't let's distract the doctor too much,' said Jill and proceeded to do just that as the four of us crossed to a large, wooden-slatted barn fronting a concrete yard, picking our way through a flock of bantams, hens and ducks. In the short walk I was given a potted history of Miss Piggy. How the saddleback had arrived as a thin, weedy piglet, the runt of the litter, the unlucky thirteenth. It had been Alex's intention to fatten her up for the table but somehow that time never arrived. And you wouldn't believe it, but he often took her for walks on a lead. Could I imagine it? A pig on a lead? People were amazed. And she was so well behaved. Trotted to heel just like a dog. Much better than their dog – a Jack Russell – she was a bit of a handful. Nipped ankles.

Oh no I thought. Not another Chico.

'No, don't worry,' Jill went on seeing me look round anxiously. 'I've shut Trisha in the house for now.'

As we reached the barn door, Emily pulled at Jill's sleeve. 'Can we watch?'

Jill looked at me, eyebrows raised.

'Don't see why not,' I said. So we all trooped in.

Miss Piggy was in a makeshift farrowing crate – a DIY job of wooden pallets tied together.

'I'm definitely not happy about her,' stated Jill, leaning over the top while Joshua and Emily peered through the gaps.

'She doesn't go "Oink" any more,' said Joshua, solemnly.

'No,' agreed Jill. 'She's gone very quiet. It's not at all like her.'

'Oink, oink,' murmured Emily pushing her arm through and poking Miss Piggy's belly.

'Now then Emily, don't,' said Jill pulling her away. 'Miss Piggy's not feeling well. You mustn't upset her.'

Tears welled up in the little girl's eyes. 'I'm only trying to make her feel better,' she sobbed.

'That's for the doctor to do.'

Yes, indeed, if possible I thought, scrambling over the pallet wall and jumping down next to the pig, flat out in a bed of straw. When I say 'flat' she was lying there motionless but far from flat. Indeed she was enormous. Her pink, blotchy abdomen swollen. Bloated. Like an over-inflated hot-air balloon about to burst.

'Dad reckons she should have had them by now,' declared Joshua.

'By the way, I must apologize that Alex's not here,' said Jill. 'He thought Eric was coming over and decided it would be best if he made himself scarce. Something to do with their golf match last Wednesday?'

Emily interrupted, her words whistling through her teeth: 'He's gone to Tethsco's.'

'Dad hates shopping,' said Joshua, still peering down at Miss Piggy. 'But he said we were out of bacon.'

'Yes ... well,' I said. There were going to be plenty of rashers here if I didn't do something to help this pig.

'Sorry,' said Jill, shushing the children. 'She's been straining all morning,' she went on. 'But we were hesitant about calling Eric – er – you out in case we were worrying unduly.'

Conscious of three sets of eyes on me, I ran my hands over the sow's extended abdomen. But she didn't stir. Not a twitch. Only the rasping bellow-like action of her thorax. I eased my hand over the coarse, ginger hair of her flank and cautiously began to feel each teat. I knew enough of pigs to know they could turn on you without warning and I didn't fancy being flattened by several hundredweight of pork. Quietly, tentatively, I moved my hand along her mammaries, ready to spring out of the way should I need to.

'She's got lots of titties,' Emily suddenly said with a giggle.

I rolled the hot, dry skin of one between my fingers and squeezed it. A tiny drop of yellow fluid appeared at the tip – a sign that she was definitely due to farrow.

'Things don't look too good,' I muttered more to myself than to my audience. But Joshua was quick to pick up on it.

'She's not going to die, is she?' he asked, the stern expression on his face beginning to crack as his eyes glistened and his lips trembled.

Jill reached out and touched his arm. 'Mr Mitchell's going to do his best, dear.'

Joshua pulled his arm away.

I levered myself round to the sow's rear end, lifted the limp, straight tail and with a rolling action, eased a thermometer through her anal sphincter. There was not a murmur from her. But certainly one from Emily.

'What's he doing now?' she queried, her eyes wide, bulging like organ stops through her glasses.

'Taking her temperature,' explained Jill.

'You didn't put it up there when I was poorly.'

'But you're not a pig, stupid,' said Joshua, recovering his composure.

'That's yuck,' said Emily with a loud tut as she watched me pull the thermometer out and wipe it on some straw.

I stood up and turned to Jill. 'Thought as much,' I said grimly. It's 40°C – way above normal. Best if I take a look inside.'

'You can't do that,' gasped Emily. 'Trisha's indoors. She'll bite you.'

'He means "Take a look inside Miss Piggy",' explained Jill, giving Emily a hug.

'Gross,' muttered Joshua, but kept his eyes fixed intently on me as I donned a plastic glove, smeared it with grease and gently began an internal examination of the sow to the accompaniment of further exclamations of 'Gross' and 'Yuck' from both children as my arm slid in deeper. She seemed relaxed and open enough to produce a piglet even though I couldn't feel one through the warm, slippery folds of her cervix. But to judge from her massive size there was a platoonful inside just waiting for the order to pop out.

Once finished, I decided to give Miss Piggy a shot of oxytocin. 'It will help to make the womb contract,' I explained to Jill.

'Bit like an induced labour then,' she said.

Emily was listening to every word. She pulled at Jill's sleeve. 'Mummy. What's a womb?'

Jill hesitated a second, looking at me with 'Help' written on her face. 'Er ... well ... it's where ....' she faltered.

'It's where the babies lie before they come out,' I said on the spur of the moment, desperate to say something.

'Like my bed womb then,' lisped Emily, apparently satisfied.

And I've got to get them out of bed soon I thought to myself as I plunged the injection into Miss Piggy's thigh, ready to spring back over the pallets should she lurch to her feet. But no. She gave only the merest of grunts, the merest twitch of her leg.

'Right,' I declared with more confidence in my voice than I felt. 'Let's give that a few hours to work.' I glanced at my watch. 'I've got evening surgery coming up. But I'm on duty afterwards. So I'll pop out later this evening.'

'Well if you're sure,' said Jill. 'That's very kind of you.'

'Mummy ... Mummy,' chorused Joshua and Emily. 'Can we stay up to watch.' They saw her shake her head.

'Oh please,' said Joshua.

'Pleathe,' echoed Emily.

'It could be way past your bedtimes.'

And it was. Well, at least there was no sign of the children when I returned that evening. The dusk of midsummer had begun to settle over the Downs, a rim of gold in the west, the outlines of the bungalow and barn blurred in an amber glow. There was a car in the drive which I guessed was Alex's. Good. An extra pair of hands would be helpful. Not so helpful was the yapping bundle of ghostly white which shot across the darkening yard, heading straight for my feet.

A head poked out of the barn door. 'Trisha. Come here you stupid mutt,' commanded a gruff voice. To no avail. The Jack Russell continued to dance and prance round my heels like a banshee on booze, only kept at bay by judicious swinging of my black bag. 'Sorry about Trisha,' apologized Alex, introducing himself. 'She's a great ratter, but when it comes to people she's a pain in the backside.'

If she could jump that high it would be another area to guard I thought, as I squeezed mine through the barn door, keeping the snapping terrier out. As a golfing buddy of Eric's I'd already formed a mental image of Alex – a similar rotund figure – both of them bouncing down the freeway together. Not a bit of it. He was a small wiry chap with something of the gypsy about him – maybe it was the dark complexion and equally dark eyes and eyebrows topped by a tangle of coal-black hair – but more likely the large gold ring looped in his left earlobe. Some sort of statement no doubt. It somehow didn't go with a 1950s' bungalow, PVC conservatory and a round of golf with Eric. But who was I to say? Me with my Calvin Klein boxers, a gold stud in each ear and an aviary full of budgerigars in my back garden.

Jill was wiping strands of sticky afterbirth from a highly vocal piglet. 'Her first,' she said, proudly holding up the shiny, pink, wriggling baby.

'Whoops … looks like her second's arriving,' exclaimed Alex. Miss Piggy gave a grunt, her balloon flanks contracting, her hindlegs stretching out; then out plopped a piglet.

'And here comes her third,' I remarked, as another shot out.

The sow showed no interest in her offspring despite their high-pitched clamour – a cacophony of squeals loud enough to engender a rush of maternal instinct in the most boorish of mothers. Not so in Miss Piggy. She just lay there, limp, exhausted, head arched back in the straw, emitting the occasional feeble grunt.

'I'll recheck her temperature,' I said, as another piglet emerged to lie spreadeagled with its litter mates.

Alex switched on an overhead lamp and angled it round to shine down on Miss Piggy's rear. As he did so another porker appeared. Her fifth. The sixth arrived seconds later.

"Must be the light attracting them,' joked Alex. But the smile belied the tension in his face.

The seventh was born as I twisted the thermometer round to read it. 39°C. Only a little less than earlier and still way above what it should be. No wonder she looked so ill.

'I reckon she's got septicaemia,' I said, raising my voice above the frenzy of squeaks. 'That's why there's no milk.' As I spoke, another three piglets joined the hungry chorusline. A protesting litter of ten were now pulling furiously on Miss Piggy's unyielding teats.

'What on earth are we going to do with this lot,' said a dismayed Jill as Miss Piggy gave another grunt and produced her eleventh and twelfth.

'Feed them, that's what,' said Alex pushing back a lock of hair. 'I'm sure we can do it.'

'You'll certainly have your work cut out,' I warned, and instantly regretted what I said. It sounded so obvious, so – what was the word

– boorish? And to judge from the dark look flashed at me by Alex he thought so too.

'At least with the weekend ahead we can have a good crack at it,' he said. 'And we can rope in Emily and Joshua to help. They'll love to.'

Jill turned to me. 'We've some milk powder in our emergency stores. Will that be OK to use?'

'Fine. Yes,' I replied. 'But add some extra glucose if you've got any … at least for the first twenty-four hours.'

'Assuming we can get it down them, how often should they be fed?'

'Ideally every two hours.'

Jill didn't bat an eyelid. 'We've a baby's bottle. Will that do?'

I nodded. 'And I've got a fostering kit in the car that you can borrow.' I didn't envy the Rymans feeding twelve young piglets but they seemed a determined couple and keen to have a go. Before I left, I gave Miss Piggy a massive intramuscular injection of long acting antibiotic in the hope that it would check the infection and bring the temperature down. Even with such a thick, viscous suspension being pumped into her leg, she showed no reaction. Not one flinch.

I suggested calling in again the following Wednesday, unless any problems cropped up before then.

'Good planning,' whispered Beryl on the Monday, giving me a conspiratorial wink with her glass eye. 'That's Crystal's morning off. She won't know anything about it.' I wondered whether she was going to enter the visit on the computer in some sort of cryptic code but decided to leave that to her. As for Eric, he pulled me into the dispensary to ask how things had gone. 'Good. Good,' he said in a low voice when I told him that Miss Piggy had farrowed. He poked his head out of the door as I mentioned the pig's fever, nervously looking up and down the corridor. What was he looking for? A spy in the camp? Tell-tale Lucy or Mandy the mole perhaps?

'I appreciate you keeping all of this under wraps,' he said, stepping back in. 'Makes it so much easier for me.'

On the Wednesday morning I found I'd been given a visit to see a Mr Myarn – an anagram of Ryman as Beryl was to explain later – clever eh?

'Yes, Myarn … you know,' said Beryl, giving me a warning look as Mandy marched through reception.

And when my morning appointments had finished, she dashed down to my consulting-room to say the coast was clear should I want to make a run for it now. What was it with this woman? Had she been watching too many reruns of *The Great Escape*? Nevertheless, I dashed out to the car resisting the urge to duck in case a hail of bullets erupted from the hospital.

'So how are things?' I asked, staring down at Miss Piggy, her family clustered round her, while the Ryman family clustered round me. 'We've managed to feed the piglets,' said Alex. 'They're fine.'

'That's my one,' said Emily pointing to the fattest and reddest. 'She's called Pinky.'

'Mine's the one kicking his legs,' said Joshua.

That must be a Perky I thought.

'We're still worried about Miss Piggy,' said Jill. 'As you can see, she hasn't really moved. No interest in food. We've tried all sorts of things to tempt her.'

I could see the trough alongside, full of untouched pellets. And on top a row of Smarties and a pile of crisps. Bacon flavoured, I wondered? Now. Now. That was naughty. This was serious.

'Are you going to stick that thing up her bottom again?' asked Emily.

There were more giggles and groans of disgust as I did so. But the temperature had dropped back to normal. I could see no reason why Miss Piggy shouldn't be on her feet. And I told the Rymans this.

'She's just a lazy cow then,' said Alex.

'She's a pig not a cow, Daddy,' said Emily crossly.

I picked up Pinky. 'You've been looking after her very well, Emily,' I said, holding up the fat little piglet. It squealed and wriggled in my hand like an animated sausage. Pork sausage of course.

Miss Piggy jerked her head up, her piggy grey eyes staring at me. All of a sudden there was a whirlwind of straw, bedding flying everywhere, a scrabbling of trotters, shrieks and squeals, one dropped Pinky, and me frantically vaulting the pallets as Miss Piggy reared to her feet and lunged at my fast disappearing legs.

As I crumpled in a heap at their feet, the Rymans leapt up and down with glee, Alex hugging Jill, a squealing Emily wheeling round in circles, arms outstretched – even serious Joshua was jigging, a broad grin etched on his face. The cause of such merriment was Miss Piggy who, as I got to my feet, remained standing on hers; with snout swinging from side to side, she swept away the straw, tracking down her scattered offspring , and drew them to her with a series of deep grunts. When her piglets were gathered round her, she gave another maternal 'Oinck', tossed aside the Smarties and crisps and buried her snout in the trough of pig nuts.

When the Rymans finally stopped their tribal dance and calmed down, it was Jill who spoke. 'Wonderful, absolutely wonderful. We can't thank you enough....' Her voice trailed off as it seemed, unusual for her, she became lost for words.

Then Emily started skipping around singing, softly at first and then louder:

'Our Miss Piggy goes Oinck ... Oinck ... Oinck,

Oinck ... Oinck ... Oinck,

Oinck ... Oinck ... Oinck.'

Jill joined in.

'Our Miss Piggy goes....'

'Oinck ... Oinck ... Oinck,' sang Alex.

'Oink ... Oinck ... Oinck,' I think I heard Joshua mutter, shoulders hunched, hands stuffed in his pockets. Certainly his lips were moving.

Miss – or rather Mrs as the Rymans now decided to call her – Piggy continued to munch without so much as an 'Oinck' of her own – but all day long.

When I returned to Prospect House, I half-expected Beryl to be in full Nazi uniform, sporting a pencil moustache. Of course she was just in her standard uniform of black trousers and long-sleeved black top; though there seemed to be a dark shadow on her upper lip, but that could just have been a trick of the light.

She immediately spotted the parcel I was carrying under one arm, its contents wrapped in a white carrier bag. I could see she was dying to ask what it was.

I wasn't going to tell her just yet. 'Spoils of war,' I said mysteriously. 'From the enemy lines. Just need to pop it in the fridge for the time being.' That had been my plan. But I hadn't thought it through properly. Nor predict the consequences of what could happen in the event of it being discovered – or rather uncovered.

The fridge was home to the vaccines and the cartons of milk used for coffee and tea. It was inevitably going to be opened several times during the course of the afternoon. And we are all curious. So I should not have been surprised that when four o'clock came and we were in the office having tea, everyone present – Crystal, Eric, Beryl and me – knew the bag contained a large hand of pork, and that everyone had read the attached ticket inside saying *Many thanks from the Rymans*. I daresay Mandy and Lucy also knew but they were down in the prep room having their break separately.

Crystal was the first to mention it, addressing Eric from behind the desk as she did so. 'You didn't tell me the Rymans had had a problem.'

Eric's mug twitched in his hand, tea slopped over the side.

'It was their sow ... Miss Piggy.' He shuffled his feet and scraped his chair back a little from the desk.

'What was wrong with her?' Crystal leaned forward, elbows either side of her mug, hands folded above it.

Eric seemed to flinch. 'A difficult farrowing, I believe.'

Crystal's eyes narrowed. 'You believe?' She sat up straight; her hands parted; her fingertips formed a pyramid.

I almost felt the urge to say 'My Lord' and come to Eric's defence. Beryl was agog, a jury of one, her head twisting from Crystal to Eric as each of them spoke.

'Well, yes it was. A difficult farrowing,' admitted Eric. He gave me a pleading look.

Now what part did I play in this little drama? If anything I was piggy-in-the-middle. Did I now save his bacon or my own?

But I needn't have worried. Crystal's customary shrewdness and ability to suss out a situation seemed to be completely out of kilter on this occasion, possibly due to lack of evidence. I could thank Beryl for that. Crystal assumed Eric had successfully dealt with the case and that the hand of pork was intended for them. 'The Rymans cure their own pork,' she said, as an aside to me. 'And very good it is too. Maybe you'll get the chance to try some one day.'

For once, despite those gorgeous eyes, I didn't feel like skipping up a mountain with her – more like pushing her over the side.

Later, as I was just about to leave, Eric expressed his thanks.

'You saved my bacon,' he said. 'Much appreciated.' He patted the plastic bag under his arm. 'Sorry about this. But if it's any consolation, it's a side of Hogmanay.'

'Hogmanay?'

'Miss Piggy's brother. Had to treat him for foot-rot not so long ago. Alex said he'd be next in line for the chop. I reckon he'll be tough as old boots.' He chuckled. 'Least it will give Crystal something to chew over.'

Yes, indeed. Oh yes, indeed. *Odl lay hee hee.*

Chapter 10

The basic routines at Prospect House continued without too many
interruptions. I accepted one never knew from day to day what
illnesses, accidents and distraught owners might alter the pattern of
those routines. Certainly the Wednesday morning for Crystal's
tennis and the afternoon for Eric's golf remained sacrosanct. Tuesday
mornings continued to be kept by for Crystal's ops. And Beryl
masterminded the appointments to ensure Crystal saw her specials
and anyone else Beryl thought merited Crystal's kid-glove approach.
Eric and I were left to mop up the rest – the rubber-glove end.

Despite Beryl's control over appointments, it didn't always work
out the way she would have liked. One Wednesday morning she was
definitely overwhelmed. Star-struck. In awe. Completely bedazzled.

'Paul, you'll never guess,' she crowed, flying into the prep room
where I was discussing the morning's list of spays and castrations with
Mandy, having finished my appointments earlier than anticipated.
'I've got the actress from that TV series up in reception. Insisting she
been seen.' She saw my blank face. 'You know … what's her name....'
She flapped her hands and tutted with exasperation. 'Oh you'll know
her when you see her.'

Oh really, I thought. Who said I was seeing her?

Mandy dropped the pack of swabs she was holding. 'I'm going to
take a peek,' she said, bumping into Lucy just as she was entering the
room. 'Hey, Lucy, we've got someone from TV up in reception,' she
said, her voice already sounding star-struck.

'Oooh I'll come as well then,' said Lucy and the two of them
rapidly elbowed each other out of the room leaving Beryl to dance
around the prep table.

'Her name's on the tip of my tongue,' she said. 'I'm sure you'll
recognize her.'

'I shall?'

'Yes ... I think she'd like to be seen now. And as you finished your appointments early today I thought you'd jump at the chance. You know, rub shoulders with someone famous. It's Crystal's morning off otherwise I'm sure she would have seen her,' she added pointedly.

'Whoever she might be,' I said drily.

'It will come to me. I can picture her now. I'm sure she was in one of those costume dramas on BBC.'

'*Pride and Prejudice?*'

'Is that the one where that chap walks out of the lake, his breeches dripping wet?'

'Yes. That was a great series. Very well done. I really enjoyed it.'

'She was in that then?'

'No she wasn't.'

'*The Mayor of Casterbridge?*'

'No.'

'*Vanity Fair?*'

'Never saw that one.' Beryl clasped her chin. 'It's on the tip of my tongue.' Several classics later and running out of titles I was still none the wiser and was about to give up when she said: '*Beat the Clock.* That was it.'

'What?'

'She used to be on *Sunday Night at the London Palladium* with that ... er ... Bruce Forsythe.'

'But Beryl, that was ages ago.' I could vaguely remember my parents used to watch it in the 60s. Besides, that had been a variety show – certainly not a costume drama. I pointed this out.

'So?' Beryl fired a look at me that could have stopped a charging rhino in its tracks. 'It was still a series.'

It's nice not to argue. To argue's not nice. So I didn't say a word.

When Mandy and Lucy returned they looked disappointed. Neither had recognized the woman though Mandy thought she might have seen her in an advert for cat food but wasn't sure.

Whatever, this so-called celebrity of Beryl's was clearly not A list, more Z by the sound of it. Though when I went up to reception to meet her, the act she put on suggested she thought she was way above the likes of those who advertised cat food even if it was top quality, came wrapped in silver foil and was fit for a queen.

'Darling,' she drawled, in a mid-Atlantic accent, an arm flamboyantly flung out to greet me as she strode across reception. 'If you could see me now I'd be so ... so grateful.' It was so ... so very Katherine Hepburn that I half expected her to have a leopard on a lead as the actress did in *Bringing Up Baby* when co-starring with Cary Grant. Now that would have been something. I could picture the headlines in the *Westcott Gazette*. YOUNG VET TREATS LEOPARD OF FAMOUS ACTRESS. Not that I considered myself a Cary Grant: more a *Carry on* – a Sid James sort.

'I'm Francesca Cavendish,' the woman was saying. 'You may have seen something of me on TV.'

A woman on a sofa with a leopard – sorry – a cat, purring round her legs waiting for her to open a pouch of tuna. Yes. Maybe I had.

This Francesca Cavendish was certainly theatrical in appearance, though the vibrant clashes of colours and styles made her, to my mind, more pantomime dame than theatrical one. The crimson, blue and yellow turban, from which a cowlick of blue and grey hair hung across her forehead could have come from Ali Baba; the purple corduroy breeches were very Prince Charming; and the brown leather boots laced to the knees echoed Dick Whittington. It was difficult to place an age on her. Beryl had reckoned on seeing her in *Beat the Clock*, and I guessed the woman was still trying to do just that – arrest the march of time. Her face was wrinkle-free, no loose chins, the skin drawn taut over prominent cheekbones as if it had been gathered up in a knot and tied beneath her turban. The porcelain features were given further doll-like attributes by ruby-red lips, the large bottom one of which constantly dropped down, and long, false eyelashes that fluttered like bats' wings at me.

Beryl had bustled back in and was now tapping details into the computer. Francesca Cavendish gave an address in Belgravia, London. 'I'm just down here for the summer,' she explained, pushing back the loop of a blue pashmina shawl that hung from her shoulder. 'Resting.'

Beryl insisted on having her 'resting' address which was a block of flats behind the multistorey car-park off Westcott's seafront.

Cat ads finished then, I thought. Now, now, put your claws away, Paul.

'So you will see me?'

'I can squeeze you in.'

'So kind.' The bats' wings gave another frenzied flap. 'I'll just get the chauffeur to bring my Oscar in then.'

What? An Oscar? Was this actress more talented than I'd imagined. Francesca Cavendish turned and gracefully floated across to the open front door, her ends of her pashmina billowing behind her. Here she paused, hand on her hip, and beckoned. A minute or so later, a man appeared carrying a dog that looked like a small fluffed-up cushion. It was a bundle of white, silky-haired, from which peered two button-black red-rimmed eyes. Not quite the Oscar I'd had in mind. I recognized the man as being the taxi driver who'd brought me up from the station for my interview. He looked at me and winked as he handed the dog over to Miss Cavendish.

'If you'd be so good as to wait in the car, I'm sure this won't take long,' she said to him, giving Oscar a kiss on the head as she gathered up the dog in her arms, enfolding him in one end of the shawl.

'If you'd like to come this way,' I said, resisting the urge to bow and point down the corridor with bent elbow whilst apologizing for the lack of a red carpet.

In the consulting-room, Francesca Cavendish billowed to a halt in front of the table and ran a finger along its surface, her bottom lip seesawing up and down as she then inspected her finger, rubbing it with her thumb.

'You can put Oscar down if you wish,' I said. 'It's perfectly safe. He won't catch anything.'

'I'd prefer to hold on to him if you don't mind,' she replied with a sniff. 'One can't be too careful. You hear of MRSA and all that in our hospitals. I dread to think what Oscar could pick up.' She gave the wrapped bundle a squeeze. She glanced about the room, her eyes alighting on my degree certificate framed on the wall. 'Yours?' she queried.

I nodded.

She studied it for a moment. 'Says you qualified this year.'

I nodded again.

'So your experience is somewhat limited then.'

Ouch. What could I say? I knew precisely what I would have liked to have said but this puss-meat Cavendish would certainly not like to hear it. Instead, I cleared my throat softly before speaking. 'So what can I do for you.'

'Darling boy, it's not what you can do for me but what can you do for Oscar here.'

Wow. I don't know about beating the clock but my ticker certainly started beating extra to the minute. It was pounding in my chest. I smiled wanly and leaned across the table, endeavouring to spot the dog, lost in layers of pashmina. I'd heard her tell Beryl that Oscar was a Maltese terrier, five years old, doctored, with a sensitive disposition and wary of men. Great. All I could see was a head – silky white hair tied over it in a blue bow matching the colour of the shawl, button-black eyes, and lips that drew back in a snarl the closer I leaned. The snarl revealed an undershot jaw with a line of yellow teeth like a row of rotting palings just waiting to impale me with their own mix of MRSA. Miss Cavendish seemed oblivious to the dribble seeping into her pashmina.

'So what seems to be the problem?' I asked.

'That's for you to find out, sweetie,' she drawled.

Tick … tick went my cardiac clock, ever faster.

'My usual vet is Mr Scott-Thomas up in Bayswater,' she went on. 'Such a nice man. Very experienced. Very understanding. His son is a casting director for TV reality shows like *Wenches in the Wilderness* and *Cast Adrift in the South Pacific* – that sort of thing. I've been approached you know.'

Not wishing to rock her boat, I feigned interest while wishing I could cast her off my premises and get her to sail in the direction of Bayswater and Scott-Thomas senior. But as Miss Cavendish pointed out, it was rather a distance to travel and for something so trivial … something she thought a provincial vet should be able to deal with. And if it turned out to be something more serious then of course she'd have no hesitation in breaking her 'rest' and taking Oscar back up to London.

Having listened to all this, I reached out to pat Oscar's head with the vague notion of establishing some sort of rapport. Some sort of contact. I certainly got the latter when a mouthful of teeth sunk themselves into my palm. I snatched my hand away half-expecting a shower of broken incisors to follow.

'There … there….' cooed Miss Cavendish, 'did the doctor frighten you? He's not like our nice Mr Scott-Thomas, is he? Now there's a doctor who knows how to treat us.'

I felt a red glow spread through me. Like molten lava welling up. A Mount Vesuvius on the point of erupting. It was only the sudden appearance of Lucy that stopped me from exploding.

'Sorry to interrupt, Paul, but we've got an RTA on our hands. Cynthia Paget's just rushed in with her chihuahua. He's been hit by a car.'

I looked at Miss Cavendish. 'Do you mind taking a seat a moment.

I must check this out.' I didn't wait for a reply but dashed out behind Lucy and ran down to the theatre where I found Mandy had Chico lying prostrate on the ops table, his pale little body looking lost on the vast expanse of the white surface. She'd a drip already set up, the needle waiting to be inserted. But, as I skidded to a halt, Chico's breathing was coming in rattling gasps and a trickle of blood oozed from his mouth. I lifted a lip, noted the blanched gums. The pupils of his eyes were widely dilated. Fixed. As I lifted my stethoscope to listen to his chest there was one final sigh and his ribcage dropped. A tremor twitched through his legs. His flanks quivered. Then stillness. Chico was dead.

A wave of sadness swept through me. Despite the little chap's habit of going for my ankles, he'd been a good companion for Mrs Paget. She was going to miss him terribly.

'Do you want me to tell her?' volunteered Mandy.

'No,' I replied. 'I think I should.'

I found Mrs Paget sitting in reception, Beryl's arm around her. She looked up, eyes red and swollen, her face streaked with tears, a handkerchief balled in her fist.

'He's gone, hasn't he?' she whispered.

I nodded. 'I'm so sorry,' I said, putting a hand on her shoulder. 'There was nothing we could do to save him.'

Mrs Paget let out another heart-wrenching sob. 'Can I see him please?'

It was Beryl who intervened. 'Yes, of course, Cynthia. You just wait here a minute.' She got up, her eyes also glistening with tears. 'I'll see to it, Paul. You've got that actress woman still to deal with.'

'Sure?'

'Yes, sure. Go on,' she insisted, giving me a slight push in the direction of the consulting-room.

Francesca Cavendish rose to her feet as I entered. 'Darling, how dreadful,' was her response when I told her of Chico's demise. Did I detect some sympathy there? But that soon evaporated when I instructed her to put Oscar on the table. Take one. Scene one. Action.

'You sure it's clean, darling? I don't want Oscar catching a nasty bug.' Cut.

'It's disinfected between each consultation. Please put him on the table.' Take two. Action.

'The disinfectant could harm his paws. He's got very sensitive feet you know.' Cut.

I pointed. 'On the table. Please.' Take three. Action.

'He might slip and slide about.' Cut.

I clicked my fingers. 'On the table.' Take four.

Yes. This time it was in the can. Oscar was unpeeled from the pashmina and lowered onto the table. He was not a pretty sight. No film or TV role would ever be offered to this undersized specimen of a Maltese terrier with his lumpy, matted coat and pink skin confetti-scattered with scurf. He immediately started bucking about the table like a pantomime horse on speed. Miss Cavendish swept him up into her pashmina again and said, 'You'll have to manage with me holding him.'

'Let's start again then, shall we? What seems to be the problem?'

This time a straight answer was given. 'He can't walk properly.'

'He's lame?'

'That's my idea of someone who can't walk, sweetie.'

Oh dear. We were off again. Must be the artistic temperament. Or just plain rudeness. Whatever, I chose to ignore it. 'So which leg's he lame on?'

There was a theatrical shrug of the shoulders. 'I'm no vet.'

Keep calm, Paul. Keep calm. I walked round the side of the table and held out my hand. 'May I?' I said, indicating the pashmina with the yellow teeth sticking out of it.

'If you insist.'

'I do.'

'Very well then.'

There was a snarl – one that emanated from Oscar rather than Francesca Cavendish – as I slid my hand into the folds of the shawl and eased out Oscar's front paws. 'I'm not going to hurt you,' I murmured.

'My dear, he doesn't know that,' she said, as I began palpating each of Oscar's toes gingerly. He fidgeted and squirmed but didn't cry out. I eased myself around the actress and levered out his hindlegs from behind her elbow. The dog whimpered as I felt his right back paw.

'Oh my sweetheart. Is he hurting you?' exclaimed Miss Cavendish with a toss of her turbaned head.

But at least I had located the problem. A dew-claw, grossly over-grown, had curled round on itself to dig into the pad. No wonder Oscar was lame. It must have been like walking on a needle. There followed a tussle between nail clippers, Maltese terrier, fingers, folds of pashmina and loose incisors as I delved into the folds of the shawl to extract paws and one by one cut nails and prise out the worst of fur balls between toes. It was a masterful performance, itself worthy of an Oscar nomination if not the statuette itself.

Nail clippings shot in all directions. Ping. One ricocheted off a steel kidney dish. Ping. Another hit a slat of the Venetian blinds. A third sprang away from the clippers and spiralled up to land ping-less in the curl of hair over Francesca Cavendish's forehead where it hung like some New Age adornment – she, oblivious to its presence.

The struggle to hang onto Oscar as he slithered and slipped out of grasp in the folds of her pashmina took their toll on the actress. By the time I'd finished, her porcelain complexion was as white and shiny as a well-scrubbed washbasin.

'Goodness,' she spluttered between gulps of air. 'I never used to have that sort of struggle with Mr Scott-Thomas.'

I refused to dwell on the image conjured up in my mind – her and him thrashing about on the consulting table. No. Definitely not. It didn't bear contemplating. I wheeled her out as quickly as I could, expressing my wish that all would now be well and that the 'rest' of her stay in Westcott would be enjoyable. I didn't suggest, as I normally did with other clients, that she should return if further problems were encountered. This one-act play with her had been quite enough. No encores were required, thank you very much.

To my surprise even Beryl, not usually one to pass judgement on clients, seemed to be on my side when she said, 'Remind me not to buy her brand of cat food.'

It must have been about ten days later when I received the call. It was one of those rare weekends where Lucy and I hadn't managed to synchronize our time off together. I was on duty; she was off; the phone at Prospect House manned by Mandy.

'Sorry, Paul,' she said, 'but I've had that pussy-ad woman on the phone demanding that her Oscar be seen.'

'Did she say what the problem was?'

''Fraid not.'

I sighed. 'Well I suppose I'd better see her then. Ask her to come in.'

'She won't.'

'What?'

'She's insisting on a house call.'

'Some hope. Especially on a weekend.'

'Maybe you could have a word?'

Minutes later I was listening to Francesca Cavendish's dramatic drawl down the line. 'You really must come out, darling. Oscar's scratching himself to death.'

'I'll certainly see him for you. But you'll need to bring him up to the hospital.'

There was a sharp intake of breath and the phone went dead.

I shrugged and put it down. 'Just that actress from the cat ads,' I said, when asked by Lucy who it was. 'Wants a house call.'

She agreed with me that the woman was unlikely to find any vet in the area prepared to make an out-of-hours visit to a scratching dog.

'But no doubt she'll ring round to try and find someone,' I said.

When the phone rang again half-an-hour later, it was Mandy to tell me that Francesca Cavendish was very sorry that we'd been cut off and what time did I say I could see Oscar?

She arrived at Prospect House before me and was sitting in the waiting room with Oscar clutched to her bosom. There was no sign of her 'chauffeur' outside. She leapt to her feet as I walked in.

She gushed, 'So good of you to see me out-of-hours.'

I forced a smile. 'No problem.'

'It's why I think so highly of Mr Scott-Thomas. However late at night it might be, he's always there for me.'

My smile faded.

'It's just that I can't stand it any longer. He's been going at it all night long. I'm quite exhausted.'

I did a double take. Had I missed something here? Some all-night hanky-panky with her Mr Scott-Thomas?

She continued: 'Scratch. Scratch. Scratch. Oscar simply won't stop. I just hope you can do something about it.'

Right. Yes. 'It must be very irritating,' I said only aware of the pun I'd made once it had slipped out. Thank goodness Miss Cavendish didn't notice. She was far more concerned at pointing out the oozing matt of fur over Oscar's right shoulder.

"Just what might that be?' she asked.

'Eczema,' I replied.

'ECZEMA?' she echoed in a tone worthy of Lady Bracknell's exclamation – 'A Handbag?' Had she been practising the part I wondered? Certainly her and Oscar looked wild enough.

My turn to take centre-stage. I explained it was wet eczema brought on by something which had irritated the skin in that region. The dog had started nibbling the spot, making it worse, more sore; so that it, in turn, made him lick more, making it even more sore so that he—

'Yes, yes, I get the picture,' butted in Miss Cavendish, waving faintly at me to stop. 'So what do you propose doing about it?'

I showed her by clipping away the wet hair and smoothing in some anti-inflammatory cream. As I did so, a small, dark-brown insect hopped across the area.

'Ah ... ah,' I trumpeted. 'There's our culprit. A flea.'

'A FLEA?'

Oh dear. Another blast of Bracknell. At this rate she'd be practice-perfect before the end of the consultation.

'How dare you suggest Oscar's got fleas.' The tone remained very Bracknell. Very Wilde. 'The very thought of it fills me with ... with....' Francesca Cavendish pounded her chest obviously searching for the appropriate dramatic expression of her disgust. Loathing? Horror? Abhorrence? Repugnance? The list was endless. But it seemed she was so choked with whatever she was filled with that the words failed to form; she just stood there, her lower lip doing its customary ventriloquist-doll-like jerking up and down, while her hand continued to beat her breast.

She finally managed to compose herself. 'Show me,' she demanded. 'The evidence. I want to see it with my own eyes.'

I parted some of the fine white hairs over Oscar's back, down by his rump. With his pink skin, it was easy to spot the black flecks I'd been searching for. I picked out several and placed them carefully on the table.

Miss Cavendish leaned over and peered down at them. 'If those are fleas why aren't they moving?' she said.

'They're not fleas,' I said, dampening some cotton wool and squeezing a few drops of water onto the flecks. Streaks of red began to spiral out. 'There's your proof,' I said. 'Flea dirts.'

Francesca Cavendish reeled back, a whole Thesaurus-ful of disgust and loathing on her face. 'That's absolutely hideous,' she said.

Hideous? Uhm. Yet another descriptive term. And yes, it certainly highlighted her feelings. As for her dog's feelings – his itchy, scratchy feelings, a couple of anti-inflammatory injections would ease those. With the first jab given, Miss Cavendish snatched the anti-flea preparation I gave her and promised to return within the week for Oscar's second injection.

'She'll have to be told,' said Lucy.

'I know. I know.' But I was dreading it. How on earth could I tactfully tell the woman the fleas weren't living on Oscar – that they only hopped on to feed?

'You'll just have to be direct,' said Lucy. 'Take the lead.'

'That's all very well,' I moaned. 'But I'm no Clarke Gable. She'll be gone with the wind if I tell her that her apartment's infested with fleas.'

But it was more like *Some Like It Hot* when I told Francesca Cavendish. She went puce. She boomed, 'You're telling me my apartment's contaminated?'

'In a manner of speaking—'

'Out with it boy. Yes or No.'

'Yes.'

There was a sharp intake of breath. A theatrical pause. 'I blame the previous tenants,' she suddenly said. 'They must have had a dog. That's how the place got infested. And to think my poor little innocent walked straight into it. Seems most likely, don't you agree, sweetie?'

Of course I was going to agree. Anything to persuade her to have the apartment treated. If she thought she wasn't the guilty party, it made it all so much easier. Indeed she was more than happy to follow my instructions. Yes. She'd thoroughly vacuum the carpets. She did that routinely anyway.

'Of course,' I murmured.

And yes. There was no problem in washing Oscar's bedding. Well, her bedding, actually – her duvet and pillows, as he slept with her. But then that was always done once a week.

'Of course.'

And spraying the entire flat with the long-acting flea spray would be no problem.

'Of course not.'

It was all very well scripted.

As for the pashmina. She'd grown tired of it anyway. It could go to the charity shop. But she'd send it to the dry cleaners first?

Yes. Of course. I lost my lines. Now who said that?

'Seems you've done her proud,' commented Eric, after overhearing Francesca Cavendish extol my virtues to a taciturn Beryl while paying the bill.

'I wouldn't want to put it quite like that, Eric,' I said, as visions of Mr Scott-Thomas 'doing her proud' reared in my head.

'Well, some people get very funny when they're told they've a flea problem. Take it as a personal affront. As if they're somehow dirty themselves. I'd imagine she'd be just the sort of woman to get stroppy.'

'She blamed it on the previous tenants at Wellington Court. So it made it all much easier.'

Eric slid a hand over his pate. 'Wellington Court, you say. Seem to remember I had a client there until recently. Can't recall what number it was though.'

'Twenty-eight,' said Beryl, who had been typing at the computer screen whilst eavesdropping. 'I've got it up on the screen here: Mr and Mrs Green, twenty-eight Wellington Court. Our Miss Puss-Ad is "resting" there at present.'

'They had a dog,' I said. 'Least Miss Puss ... er ... Francesca Cavendish thinks they did.'

Eric shook his head. 'Well, she's wrong. All the Greens had was a budgie. I used to clip its beak.'

He saw the look I gave him. 'Don't worry. I won't let on. But it may cost you a pint or two.'

'Done,' I declared, without a moment's hesitation. No way did I want Francesca Cavendish coming back to give me a flea in my ear. Alive or dead.

Chapter 11

Mandy, in one of her more affable moods, had warned me not to. Eric said they were a minefield. And Beryl commented it wasn't the wisest thing to consider doing. But it was Crystal who was most adamant about the dangers of being a judge at a pet show. And that surprised me as I would have thought the publicity generated for the practice would have been a good thing.

'Not so, Paul,' said Crystal, as we sat discussing the possibility one lunchtime early in August. 'Some years back I was persuaded to judge the dog classes at Westcott's August Bank Holiday Show. It was a real nightmare, believe you me.'

I tried to visualize the cool, calm collected woman sitting in front of me, not a hair out of place, her neat manicured fingers daintily folded round her bone china mug of herbal tea as being in nightmare situation. Crystal ruffled? Never.

She continued, 'The thing was I never heard the last of it from those clients who didn't win rosettes. Not that they said anything of course. It's just that for months afterwards undercurrents of resentment could be felt whenever they came into surgery. I've no wish to jeopardize the special relationship I have with my clients. So I now leave judging of shows to the practice down the road.'

So there. I had been warned. No excuse. But then I hadn't reckoned on the persuasive powers of a child to disarm me.

I'm not sure who had given my phone number. I suspected it could have been Revd Matthews from our local church in Ashton passing it on to the church in the neighbouring village. Some sort of clerical networking – I'll ring your bells if you ring mine.

The voice down the line was high-pitched, with a slight nervous tremor. A choirboy perhaps – ready to sing my praises? No. It sounded more like a girl, and one anxious to seek salvation. Straightaway, I was asked if I could judge the pet show at their church fête. 'It's just that we hadn't realized our usual vet would be away on holiday next weekend.'

Next weekend? It was Thursday now. It was hardly giving me much notice. But why should that concern me? I wasn't going to do it. The warnings from Beryl, Eric and Crystal rang in my head louder than.... 'Which church is it?' I found myself saying.

'St Augustine's in Chawcombe.' The voice sounded a little more hopeful.

Now why had I asked? I'd just told myself I wouldn't do it, so what did it matter which church it was?

'You should try one of the other vets in the area.'

There was a pause and some muffled conferring. 'We already have,' said the girl coming back on the line. 'Six, in fact.'

Six? For a brief moment I was miffed to think I was that far down the ranking of vets in the district. But come on, Paul, why worry? I wasn't going to be involved.

Yet I was unable to stop myself from asking, 'And all six turned you down?'

'Yes, they did,' said the girl, sounding decidedly weepy. 'But one tried to be helpful. He faxed us a list from the *Veterinary Register*. And we've been going through that.'

How inconsiderate those six vets had been. One of them could have volunteered. Stopped me being put on the spot.

'You're our last chance,' she went on. 'We're down to the Ws: there's no one else left on the list.'

'But I'm M: M for Mitchell,' I said. Again, did that really matter?

There was more muffled conferring. 'Thought you'd been through the Ms.' 'Have.' 'Haven't.' 'Have ... look ... see? I've ticked them off.' 'But what about him? Oh!' The voice returned. 'My sister says she's sorry but she'd overlooked you.'

Mmm. Pity it couldn't have stayed that way. 'You've done the Ws, you say?' I queried, desperately racking my brains for a way out. Wasn't there a new vet who'd just put up his plate in Westcott? Now what was the chap's name? Wilson. Yes, that was it, Wilson. Now surely he'd jump at the chance of helping out. A little bit of free advertising. A mention in the parish magazine.

'Wilson?' echoed the girl. More whispering. 'We've tried him.'

'And?' I didn't need to know the answer. He'd be working that afternoon. As it seemed were all the other vets the girl had contacted. My, my. What a busy bunch of vets we were in this part of Sussex. Especially next Saturday afternoon.

'You're not working as well, are you?' There was desperation in her voice.

As it happened I wasn't, and providing the weather remained fine I was looking forward to a leisurely afternoon in the back garden at Willow Wren soaking up the sun. But how could I do that without feeling guilty about not helping out? Besides which, it was bound to get back to Revd Matthews; with the rectory opposite Willow Wren – the other side of the churchyard – I could see me digging my own grave there if I refused.

I began to weaken. 'What sort of show is it?'

The girl's tone brightened instantly. 'It's very small.'

'Yes. But what would I be judging?' Crystal's words filled my head. The last thing I wanted were owners who thought I'd misjudged them – or rather their dogs.

'It will just be children's pets.'

That didn't sound too bad. A few mice. A handful of hamsters. The odd rabbit or two. Yes, I could handle them without too much hassle. So I agreed. 'And what time does it start?' I asked.

'Three o'clock in the vicarage garden. But I should get there early if I were you. It's usually quite popular and there's often lots of entries. So you might need extra time to judge them.'

Warning bells should have rung then. But didn't.

They started to toll when I told Mandy. Then Eric. Then Beryl. They all wrung their hands. Crystal just raised hers and shrugged her shoulders in a 'you have been warned' fashion.

'Pray for rain,' was all Lucy would say.

A large depression on the Friday lifted mine but overnight a ridge of high pressure wriggled in and Saturday dawned warm and sunny.

'There. The perfect day for a fête,' chuckled Lucy, drawing back the bedroom curtains. A shaft of sun, reflected off the church clock, beamed in and shone across the bed to hit me in the face like some lighthouse beacon picking out a wreck. I certainly felt like one. A nervous wreck.

'Oh, don't be such a namby-pamby,' exclaimed Lucy, pulling the sheet off me. 'It's only children's pets. It's not as if you'll have to contend with the likes of Miss McEwan and her mynah or that actress with her Maltese. It should be a doddle.'

Despite her reassuring words, I still hoped for some divine intervention. A plague of locusts perhaps? But us British are such a resilient lot. The show would still go on. And no doubt some bright spark would enter one of the locusts for best pet. In the end the only divine intervention I got was in the form of the gangly figure of Revd Matthews who popped over just before I left for Chawcombe. He carried a sponge cake wrapped in cellophane under one arm.

'I hear from Charles that you're going to be judging the pets this year.' Seems the evangelical hot line had clearly been in action. 'I'm so pleased for him. It's difficult to find someone each year. You vets are always so busy this particular weekend. Either that or away on holiday.'

I assumed Charles was the vicar of St Augustine's, a man whom I had yet to meet.

'Anyway,' continued Revd Matthews, 'this is just to say I hope it all goes well for you. Bless you. Oh, and the wife baked this cake this morning.' He handed me the sponge while his upper lip did its customary curl up over his teeth as he beamed.

What a nice gesture. I was a glutton for homemade cakes and was just about to thank him when he added, 'It's just a little extra for the cake stall at the fête. Susan always likes to make a contribution. Has done so for the past two years. Not that she expects to win gold three years in a row. But it's all in a good cause. And I do hope you don't run into too many difficulties in your judging. You know what people are like with their pets. These shows can turn into a bit of a bun fight. And I'm not talking cakes here.' He looked serious for a moment and patted my arm. 'But I'm sure you'll pull through. My thoughts will be with you.' He gave me another reassuring pat.

Goodness. What was all this in aid of? He made it sound as if I was being sent off to the Crusades in the Holy Land rather than off to a pet show in the next village. It did nothing for my nerves.

Nor did the congested lanes in and around Chawcombe. It seemed like the whole of West Sussex was descending on the place. And there was me thinking there'd be just a few dedicated church supporters sprinkled on the vicarage lawn.

Instead, I was forced to park nearly a mile from the church, join the throng of people streaming down the lane and queue for over five minutes at the vicarage gate where a makeshift ticket office in the form of a kitchen table and two washing up bowls had been positioned.

'That'll be a pound, mate,' declared the man at the gate, proffering me a ticket and a programme, his other hand outstretched, palm up.

'I'm ... er ... judging,' I said.

'Cakes?' He pointed to the sponge under my arm.

'Er ... no. Pets.'

'Really?' A broad grin split his weatherbeaten face. His bulbous nose wobbled and a little black bristle on the end of it jumped up and down. 'You'll have your work cut out then.'

Despite the sun burning down on my head, the heat failed to melt the ice pack that suddenly clamped my heart. Just what was I letting myself in for?

'It's at the far end of the garden,' he continued. 'You'll see a path leading down into a copse. There's a sign – "Pets' Corner". You can't miss it. You'll pass the cake stall on the way. But you'll have to be quick with that.' He nodded at the cake under my arm. 'Entries are just about to close.'

I started elbowing my way through the slowly moving throng, peering over shoulders wondering where the cake stand was. I passed a jumble stall where a swirling mass of ladies were tunnelling through the piles of clothes like ferrets in a rabbit warren. Every so often an article of possible interest was exposed with a squeal of delight, dragged out, examined and then tossed back in again with a shake of the head. Skirts, blouses and the odd shoe or two winged through the air. A buttonless military-style blouson clipped my ear and landed on my shoulder only to be snatched away by a whiskery woman who barked 'Leave off. That's mine.'

I pushed forward, squeezing through the crowd, careful to keep a protective arm across the vicar's cake tucked under my elbow. Heaven help me if something happened to that. Which in the next blur of seconds it did. There was a whining, a panting, the smell of hot doggy breath and suddenly I was clutching at nothing. The cake had slipped from my grasp, snatched from behind me and, as I swung round, was now in the jaws of a Dalmatian, jam oozing from his jowls.

'Oh, Henry ... really. You wicked dog,' admonished a woman in broad-belted, low slung jeans who came striding up behind him to yank at his equally broad-belted leather collar; an action which made the dog hack which in turn caused the sponge-turned-trifle to be spewed onto the grass where its fate was well and truly sealed by a passing sole which ground it into the grass. 'I'm so, so sorry,' she continued to says, but Henry's a glutton for cake.' Henry slobbered and pulled at his collar, looking up at me as if expecting another titbit. A slice of Madeira maybe? Date and walnut?

I muttered something along the lines of 'Not to worry' although inwardly squealing with anguish. If God worked in mysterious ways then he now had me completely baffled. This was turning into more of a chimp's tea party than a vicar's and I still had the judging to do. I stepped out of the jam – the human one spread round the jumble stall – and headed across a paved terrace at the back of the vicarage. French windows were wide open. A sign stuck to a pane of glass informed people of the teas available inside with a list of cakes on offer. Good job Henry the Dalmatian couldn't read.

A hot and flustered group of youngsters had assembled at one end of the terrace, settled themselves on chairs and were busy picking or blowing their noses in between doing the same to a variety of musical instruments. As I scooted off in my continuing search for the 'Pets' Corner' the band turned from noses to musical scores and struck up a rousing *Colonel Bogie*.

I eventually found the copse at the end of a well-tended kitchen garden, the path through the middle of which was bounded by rows of runner beans forming wigwams of green down each side. To the left along a mellow brick wall ran a lean-to greenhouse, the panes of which mirrored silver in the blistering heat.

A page torn from an exercise book and nailed to a tree trunk proclaimed 'Pets Corner' in red ink with an arrow pointing down into the glade. Stepping from the blinding light into the gloom of the copse was like stumbling into pitch-blackness. Until my eyes adjusted, I couldn't see where I was going and blindly slipped and slid down a path still tacky and wet from the thunderstorms earlier in the week. I staggered to a halt in the middle of the glade blinking like a batty barn owl. Slowly I became conscious of pairs of eyes – row upon row of them – encircling me.

To every tree was tied a dog. Several overweight black Labradors sat, bow-legged, bellies hanging down, tongues lolling out, chains of saliva dangling from their jowls. A white poodle, the red bow in its top-knot askew over one eye, was rapidly turning brown as it scrabbled in the mud grizzling for its owner. An Irish setter was trying to mount a dachshund while a boxer had tied itself in knots round a clump of holly in an attempt to take a chunk out of a growling Jack Russell.

A girl of about fourteen with long, mousy hair tied back in two bunches, picked her way over.

'Have you a pet?' she asked.

I recognized her voice as the one belonging to the girl on the phone. 'I'm Mr Mitchell.'

The girl's face remained blank.

'The vet. You asked me to judge the pets.'

'Oh, yes. Right. Well....' The girl spread her hands and looked round the glade at all the canine eyes now staring at us with intense interest.

I stared back with far less enthusiasm. 'So where are the owners?'

'I thought it best if they left their dogs tied up.' The girl gave an apologetic smile. 'It was getting so crowded and churned up down here.'

The gloom of the glade seeped into me, not helped by the mud which clung tenaciously to my shoes. Oh well, I thought, I've landed myself in this so might as well get on with it. Get some of the animals looked at before their owners return. I pulled a small notebook from my pocket and began to make notes. By my sixth identical-looking black, fat, middle-aged Labrador I was getting confused. There must have been some fertile Chawcombe bitch churning out such puppies like peas from a pod.

I turned to the poodle which now resembled a brown rat, bow adrift, paws so caked in mud that she had difficulty in lifting them. But she had no problem in lifting her lip as I bent down to examine her – an action which had her immediately struck off my list of possible finalists.

I approached the boxer. He strained forward on his leash, wagged the stump of his tail furiously, blustering and spraying saliva like a leaking hosepipe.

'Well, boy, you seem pleased to see me,' I exclaimed, ruffling his ears as his rump continued to thump from side to side against my legs. Yes, you could be a finalist I decided and was marking him down when I felt my left trouser leg go warm and soggy. I wheeled round to find the boxer's leg cocked against mine, a jet of urine still squirting out.

'Why, you dirty bugger!' I exclaimed, jumping out of range. One less for the list.

By now people were beginning to trickle back in, the trail taken becoming more and more treacherous the more people that came down it. A slippery slope that was crying out for an accident to occur. But it took the arrival of several more entries – two rabbits, a goldfish, some furry things in cages – before it happened. A short, buxom lady suddenly filled the entrance to the glade, her rounded bulk silhouetted against the sky. I could just make out the box she was holding in her arms. It was covered in a raised layer of chicken-wire from which peered a row of ginger kittens – three in all, each emitting a chorus of plaintive miaows. Dragging his heels behind her was a boy of about five, and it was his heels that brought both her and his downfall. He slipped on the slope, caught his foot in a tree root and grabbed at his mother's T-shirt to stop himself falling. She was jerked back, her legs jerked forward and both she and the boy landed on their backs and skidded down the slope. The box sailed into the air, the mesh springing off to the right the kittens springing out to the left.

The effect was like a dam bursting. The glade erupted in a swell of howls, barks, hisses and spits interspersed with a torrent of swear words as more owners poured in to cascade down the path and flood the glade, awash now with dogs leaping and twisting on their leads, a sea of canines tying themselves and their owners in knots.

Mortified, I shrank back against a tree, my hands clawing at the trunk behind me as if it were a life-raft. Could this really be happening? When I heard the band strike up *Bare Necessities* from the film *Jungle Book* I began to wonder whether Mowgli would suddenly appear in the glade with Baloo the bear waltzing down behind him wanting to be judged Best Pet. Nonsense. It was my imagination running wild, not the glade. Though that gorilla of a man shambling across the clearing did look like King Louie. And that hissing sounded more Kaa, the cobra, than cat.

When things eventually settled down, the kittens recaptured, my notepad retrieved from the mud and wiped down by the girl, I had no option but to get on with the judging.

'Phoebe wouldn't hurt a fly,' remonstrated the platinum-permed owner of the white-brown poodle. She, like her pet, had a red bow in her hair and matching white-trousered legs muddied up to the calves. Phoebe confirmed her position at the bottom of my list by baring her rotten teeth at me as I edged past.

'Fine example of her breed, don't you think?' boomed the gorilla-owner of the red setter. I'd seen this King Louie before. No. Not in *Jungle Book* but somewhere in Westcott. Now, just where was it? Ah, yes. Of course. The dental practice. I'd gone there last week to register. He was the gorilla (dentist) who'd swung over the chair to check my teeth and found a cracked filling. He'd put in a temporary one while making a template for a ceramic replacement. I was due back next week. Lucas was his name. And, yes, I'm sure he recognized me.

'So what do you say?' he asked, his piggy yellow eyes staring hard at me before he pulled the dog over and ordered her to sit. This she did without a murmur.

I lifted her muzzle and drew back the lips on one side to inspect her teeth. The back molars were encrusted with tartar.

'Like you, she needs a bit of dental work,' Lucas confessed. 'But I guess we both know the drill.' He gave a couple of earthy grunts which could have been construed as a chuckle. I was far from amused. He of all people, being a dentist, should have known better than to allow such a build-up of tartar. Another pet to be struck off my list.

Lucas suddenly thrust his face in mine. 'You're due to come back next week, aren't you?'

'Er … yes,' I replied, letting the setter's lip drop.

'I've got to drill out that temporary filling if I remember correctly.'

'So I believe.'

'Yessss … quite a deep cavity you've got there.' There was a menacing glint in the piggy eyes. 'Could be painful. Very painful in fact.'

I couldn't believe what I was hearing. Intimidation? A veiled threat? It was enough to set one's teeth on edge – especially in my case where a replacement filling was required. I quickly reinstated the dog. Well, she was very obedient.

A little girl rammed a hamster cage in my stomach.

'He's called Ermintrude. 'Erm for short.'

I was still mentally writhing in a dentist's chair, not concentrating. 'Gertrude. That's a nice name.'

'No, silly. Ermintrude.'

I peered through the bars. All I could see was a mound of shredded paper. 'So how long have you had Gert … er … Ermintrude?'

'Bought him this morning.'

This wasn't exactly the child-pet rapport I was seeking and decided to move on.

A gravelly voice grated in my ear. "Ere, you haven't examined him yet. Rules are rules. You need to give him the once-over.' The voice belonged to yet another portly woman whom I took to be the little girl's mother. I was also quick to note the fact that the Bastille proportions of the woman belonged to Jane Bradshaw, the sister at the health centre in Westcott. No mistaking that bulk. No liana in any jungle – even one conjured up by Kipling – could support such a massive frame as hers. This Jane swung round on me and glared. Me being no Tarzan capitulated at once, stuck my finger in the cage and had it bitten for my trouble. I swore and pulled my hand out.

'Needled you did he?' said Mrs Bradshaw.

'Sharp little fellow,' I said, nursing my punctured finger. Another pet deleted from my list.

'Couldn't do better myself,' she said. 'In fact, I could do far worse.' She fixed me with steel-grey eyes. 'Far worse. Just remember that when you next need to come in for a tetanus jab.' She emphasized 'jab' and poked my arm viciously with a finger. This was a plain Jane plainly speaking. No beating about the bush ... or jungle. The hamster rapidly reappeared on my list.

The girl with the bunches tapped me on the shoulder and asked how things were going.

'Thought you said it was only children's pets,' I hissed, feeling decidedly Kaa-like. Decidedly viperous.

'It was supposed to have been. But the printers made a mistake. The "children's" bit got left out of the programme. Still, it means we've had lots more entries,' she added brightly. 'And it's good for the church funds.' She held up a jangling money-box.

'What's your name?' shrilled a voice, slicing through the air. 'My name's Cedric.'

Oh, no. Surely not? I turned, first catching sight of the metallic cage being carried by a youth, and then the white head of Miss McEwan bobbing behind. With a nimbleness that belied her age, she zigzagged down the path and skirted the worst of the muddy patches before drawing level with me, her face lighting up the gloom with a beaming smile.

'Good afternoon, Mr Mitchell,' she twittered. 'A little bird told me you were going to be judging the show.'

Cedric no doubt, I thought glumly, as the mynah sprang up and down his perch and gave me a 'Well here I am. Aren't I a pretty boy?' look.

I glanced at my watch. It was way past three o'clock. 'Well, actually,' I said, 'the entries closed at three. We've now started the judging.'

'Oh, don't worry about that,' interjected the girl rattling the money-box under Miss McEwan's nose. 'That'll be fifty pence please.'

'Oh Lady Luck's with me today,' cried Miss McEwan, diving a hand into her bag. 'And I'm sure Mr Mitchell will think the same.'

She ordered the youth with the cage to move forward and then waved at Cedric. 'He's all yours,' said she.

'Bugger off,' said the bird.

'Now, Cedric. Naughty, naughty. Mr Mitchell doesn't want to hear that sort of language. He wants to hear how well I look after you. All those visits to the surgery. They cost me a pretty penny.'

'Pretty penny,' trilled Cedric giving me a beady look.

Miss McEwan craned her neck till her own beady eyes were level with my lapels. 'But I don't mind spending out if it warrants it. But you'll be the best judge of that, won't you, Mr Mitchell?' she added, her voice dropping several decibels to sound distinctly threatening.

'Watch it,' intoned Cedric gravely.

Oh no, I groaned inwardly. Not more intimidation. And this time from a mynah Mafia. I'd have my eyes pecked out by crows next if I didn't watch it. I could just see it … well, actually, I wouldn't if the crows got their way. As it was, I only needed the local baker to threaten to slice me up wholemeal, the grocer to give me a cauliflower ear and the butcher to make mincemeat of me and I could be driven out of Chawcombe – back to Ashton – five miles as the crows fly – providing they didn't get me first.

Keep calm, I thought. Don't be swayed. I made encouraging noises to Miss McEwan, saying how high the standard of entries was, such a variety of interesting pets, and how, of course, Cedric was extra special, no doubt worthy of being a winner. At that point, Cedric blew a loud raspberry. Mmm. Seems he wasn't such a dumb bird after all. I excused myself and turned back to the lines of pets still waiting to be judged.

By the time I'd looked at the ginger kittens, four budgerigars, two more hamsters and my eighth black Labrador, I was completely befuddled – my mind swimming in circles like the goldfish in the bowl I was now peering into.

'You've already looked at him,' said his spotty owner.

Finally, when I'd almost given up, my attention was caught by a small boy in grey flannels, some way apart from the mainstream of people, patiently standing at the edge of the glade, a slim Labrador, black of course, quietly sitting by his side. I picked my way over several intertwined leads to reach him.

'Hello. What's your name?'

'Thomas,' said the boy shyly.

'Well, Thomas, you've a nice quiet dog here.'

The boy's face creased in a frown for a moment. 'Actually, Cindy's not really mine. She's my dad's.'

'Ah, but I'm sure you help to look after her.'

'Oh, yes. I do,' said the boy with a grin. 'I'm allowed to feed her. But I have to be careful 'cos she's very greedy. Dad says she'll get too fat otherwise.'

'Do you take her for walks?' Cindy's head twisted to one side, her ears pricking up.

'Oh yes. She chases rabbits on the Downs.'

'Does she now.'

'I know she shouldn't and I do try to stop her. Honest.' Thomas put a protective arm round the Labrador's neck. 'Don't I, Cindy?' He kissed her on the head and she turned to lick his face.

I liked the rapport evident between the boy and the dog. The Labrador seemed in peak condition; shining coat, bright clear eyes, and slim – no doubt from all that rabbit chasing. Yes, I decided, Cindy would be the overall winner. Second place I'd give to a little girl's Peruvian guinea pig – a fine specimen, its hair smartly spiked in whorls of tan, black and white. And third would be an elderly border collie who spent the entire time snoozing, oblivious of the uproar around her. Whether she was well trained or just dog-tired and counting sheep I couldn't tell. But her teenage owner, despite his jeans with knees protruding and gold rings clipped in all visible orifices, seemed very fond of the old girl, and that's what counted with me.

Keeping my head down, I skirted past Mr Lucas and his red setter, side-stepped Jane Bradshaw with difficulty and tiptoed away from Miss McEwan though I didn't escape the notice of sharp-eyed Cedric who emitted an extra loud raspberry as I made my escape. I told the girl of my choice, handing her the list.

'Well, if you really think so,' she said dubiously, scanning the three names.

Puzzled at her reaction, I watched her hurry away.

The prizes were to be presented on the terrace where a space had been cleared for owners and their pets to parade. We all spilled out from the glade like battered bats, dazzled by the strong sunshine. The band struck up a discordant *All Things Bright and Beautiful* as the boxer took a chunk out of the haunch of the Jack Russell; the poodle panicked, slipped from the trouser-suited lady's arms, knocked the spotty lad's bowl from his; this sent the goldfish flying – only to be snapped up by Mr Lucas's red setter with a smack of lips while Cedric shrieked with laughter.

Just as well the fish hadn't been a prize winner.

With owners and pets lined up in front of the terrace with Miss McEwan head and shoulders below but several feet ahead of the others, the last, excruciating notes of the band faded away.

The vicar strode forward, a large benevolent smile curled across a full-moon face framed in a shock of sandy hair. 'So sorry not to have introduced myself earlier,' he whispered, shaking my hand vigorously while thrusting a mike in the other. 'But please do announce the winners.' He stepped back and stood, hands clasped behind his back, head tilted to one side, waiting.

Miss McEwan waved her purse to and fro, Mr Lucas bared his gleaming white tombstones, while Jane Bradshaw's right forefinger repeatedly jabbed the beefy biceps of her left arm.

'Well, ladies and gentlemen, it gives me great pleasure,' I said, waving the microphone inches below my chin. The Tannoy hissed and crackled feebly.

'Speak up, mate,' someone called out from the back. 'We can't hear you.'

The vicar jolted from his meditative stance and sprang behind the band. 'Is that any better?' I heard him call out.

I cleared the frog in my throat. The sound leapt out of the Tannoy like an army of frogs in jackboots. The front row visibly flinched. But I continued, saying how gratifying it was to have had so many entries – a raspberry from Cedric here – and what a high standard and how difficult it had been to decide on the three winners – another raspberry – but here were the three winners in reverse order – silence from Cedric at this point. I called out the third and second prize winners and they received their envelopes of money amidst polite applause.

'And now for the Champion Pet.' I paused for dramatic effect, keeping my eyes off the three mafiosi in front of me. 'This goes to a little lad and his Labrador, Cindy. Would Thomas Venables kindly step up.'

An audible murmur of surprise rippled through the crowd. I looked at the vicar whose mouth had dropped open, his face rapidly turning puce.

The lad emerged from the crowd and trotted up onto the terrace, Cindy trotting beside him. 'Here, Dad, could you hold onto Cindy while I collect my prize,' he said, handing the Labrador's lead to the vicar who dithered a moment before taking the dog. Cindy greeted him with a frenzied wag of her tail.

The applause was muted as Thomas received his envelope of money and I even thought I heard someone shout 'Fixed'. Certainly Miss McEwan, Mr Lucas and Jane Bradshaw didn't clap. They were mentally knifing me by the look of daggers in their eyes. And even Revd Venables had a hint of steel in the look he gave me as he bade me farewell. Clearly he was not over the moon about my decision despite the beneficent smile fixed to his face.

If I expected sympathy for my *faux pas*, I was sadly mistaken. Beryl crowed with laughter when I related the events of the afternoon. Eric bounced up and down with a chuckle. Lucy and Mandy just showed how immature they both were by rolling around, clutching themselves and howling, tears streaming down their faces.

Only Crystal showed a decent level of concern and sympathy – just as I would have expected of such a cool, calm, elegant lady.

'Poor boy,' she said, reaching out to place a hand on my shoulder, those gorgeous blue eyes of hers gazing tenderly into mine. 'What an ordeal it must have been.' Her lips started to quiver, her eyes began to glisten. 'I'm sorry, Paul ... but....' she choked. She bit her lip. A tear rolled down. There, see? She knew just how I'd felt. Any minute now, more tears of sympathy would begin to roll. And they did – in bucketloads – as, unable to fight them back, she dissolved in tears of laughter.

I got all huffy. Petulant. If she was going to act like that, well BYE-BYE Julie Andrews. See if I cared. She'd no longer be one of my favourite things.

Chapter 12

By the time summer slipped into early autumn, Lucy and I had settled into a comfortable routine of living together. We were lucky to have Willow Wren with its long, snaking back garden, the picturesque village setting and the kindly neighbours: Joan and Doug Spencer next door, and across the way, the well-meaning Revd Matthews and his wife, Susan. She'd been very understanding about the demise of her sponge. 'It was obviously not meant to be,' she'd said, casting her eyes heavenwards.

Work too was a factor which drew Lucy and I closer together. Though often hectic, chaotic, traumatic, our mutual love of animals and concern for their welfare was a common bond. If ever the pressures of working at Prospect House seemed to be reaching boiling point in one of us, the other was there to talk it through, help ease the tension, get things back on an even keel.

But in the last few weeks, there'd been something on Lucy's mind. She'd been distinctly less chirpy, more snappy, flaring up at the slightest thing. So unlike her.

'What's wrong, Luce?' I'd asked on several occasions. But each time it was met with a shrug, a 'Nothing' and a quick change of subject, or worse – a stony silence.

This afternoon was a good example. Earlier, even though I'd just got back from a busy morning surgery, I'd offered to prepare lunch. There was an Italian ready meal in the freezer which needed eating up.

'Why is it when you offer to do lunch, it's a ready meal,' she complained. Ah. Fair point, I suppose. Echoes of my days at Mrs Paget's when my time in her kitchen was strictly limited and ready meals were the only option.

'Well, I'll rustle up an omelette then,' I'd said to Lucy. We usually had a small but steady supply of eggs from Bertha and Belinda, our two Rhode Island Reds that Lucy had acquired as part of our burgeoning menagerie.

'They've just gone off-lay, in case you hadn't noticed,' she replied. 'We've no eggs unless someone bothers to go to the supermarket.' The 'someone' was clearly emphasized – the inference that it would be her yet again obvious. Tetch. Tetch. I don't know about chickens being off-lay: I was feeling distinctly hen-pecked.

Ah, yes, Paul, I remonstrated to myself. Should have looked in the fridge first. Careful now. Better watch my step – seems I might be treading on eggshells even if there aren't any eggs.

A compromise was eventually reached – spaghetti Bolognese. At least it showed more effort on my part; the spaghetti and mince needed cooking even if the sauce did come out of a jar. The meal was eaten in silence.

That silence continued during the afternoon as we took the opportunity of savouring the warmth of the September sunshine, lying on loungers in the back garden. But it did nothing to dispel the chill between us. Pity, as it really was a glorious day. One of those early autumn days, misty in the morning, a touch of mellowness in the air, a hint of gold and red in the trees and colour still in the borders. We had clumps of purple Michaelmas daisies over which the occasional red admiral flitted, a second flush of yellow roses over the back door, and a tree still laden with rosy apples, many of which had dropped and on which wasps were feeding, getting drunk on the juice.

One such inebriated insect was now spiralling over me in ever-decreasing circles, likely at any moment to land in a drunken sprawl on my head. I flicked it away. It headed across to Lucy, who was sitting a few feet from me, legs tucked under her, staring into space. She was like a coiled spring awaiting release. The tension was almost palpable.

Suddenly, she broke the silence.

'Where did that come from?'

For a moment I thought she was referring to the wasp and was tempted to say 'From the apples' but checked myself. Drunken wasps were difficult enough to cope with let alone barbed comments flying between us.

'What?' I feigned confusion. Not too difficult to do as despite the coldness emanating from Lucy, the warm sun was making me feel quite mellow – almost as mushy as the rotting apples. Certainly not waspish.

'That creature.'

'Creature. What creature?' Were we talking more wasps here? Or a bee perhaps – the one in Lucy's bonnet?

A finger was pointed at a spot below me. 'Under your lounger.'

I rolled to one side and looked under. A pair of yellow eyes belonging to a small tortoiseshell cat looked up. She cringed back as I shifted my weight. 'Why, it's a cat.'

Lucy's sunglasses had slipped down the bridge of her nose. She peered over them, her hazel eyes hard as nuts. 'You don't have to be a vet to see that.'

Ouch. I was stung and the wasp was nowhere in sight. This really wasn't the Lucy I'd fallen in love with. Just what was wrong with her?

'Well?' By the tone of her voice, winter had definitely arrived early. 'What's it doing there?'

I could have been facetious and said: 'Having a cat nap' or 'Having kittens – like me'. But such witticisms are best handled by the likes of Noël Coward and as I was feeling more coward than Noël, I decided to keep the catty comments to myself. Instead, in the best traditions of the British in times of crises, I asked Lucy if she'd like a cup of tea. It didn't work. The cat, not a cuppa, was uppermost in her mind.

'Is it one you've sneaked home from the surgery without telling me?'

I began to bridle. 'Sneaked home? Why on earth should I do that? We've enough of a menagerie here as it is with all your lot.' Whoops. That was the wrong thing to say. Even if true. Nelson, the deaf Jack Russell, the three cats, the assortment of guinea pigs, rabbits, pheasants and ferrets had all been acquired by Lucy – Gertie the goose was the only exception.

I sat up and swung my legs over the edge of the lounger. 'Look, Lucy, I had a hectic surgery this morning. A chock-a-block appointments list. The last thing I'd have felt like doing was bringing a cat home with me. OK?' I peered under the lounger again. The tortoiseshell had shrunk back even further, frightened by my raised voice. 'Perhaps it's come from next door.' That was hardly likely as Doug Spencer had told me that although he was fond of cats, his wife wouldn't tolerate them in the house. Joan did upholstery and was afraid a cat would damage her fabrics.

'I'm sorry puss, but you're not wanted,' I went on. 'So I suggest you bugger off and find somewhere else.' The cat remained crouched, back arched with no indication of moving on. 'Well, it's your choice,' I muttered, flopping back on the lounger. 'But don't expect any sympathy. It's in short supply round here at the moment.'

There was the click of sunglasses as Lucy snatched hers off, folded them and jumped up to storm indoors. I was hoping it was just a storm in a teacup. And that she'd return with just tea in a cup, but somehow I knew more than tea was brewing. If only she'd discuss what was troubling her instead of letting things stew.

'Right, the coast's clear, mate,' I said, tapping the side of the lounger. The cat slunk out and padded slowly across the patio, pausing to look back at me. She was a pretty little thing; short-haired, her coat a patchwork of golden brown, black and white with an appealing black patch over one eye and four white socks. 'Shouldn't hang around if I were you. More than your life's worth. Even if you have got nine of them. Go on, scram.' I clapped my hands and the little cat shot over the wall into the Spencer's garden. Oh dear, not the best of moves. No warm welcome there, I feared.

It was Beryl who gave me some inkling of what was troubling Lucy.

'It's to do with Mandy,' she informed me. We were sitting by the back door of Prospect House, making the most of the continuing good weather – a bonus for Beryl as it made it easier for her to smoke out in the open. On wet days she had to keep the door ajar and flick the ash out into the rain.

'Yes,' she said, watching a curl of smoke drift up into the forget-me-knot blue sky before taking another drag. 'Heard them arguing down in the prep room. Mandy was in one of her preachy moods. You know how she is sometimes.'

I did indeed, having often been subjected to her 'bossy boots' manner myself. But then she did know her stuff. And Lucy was here to learn. But obviously something was rattling her, as she went round with such a long face she could have scraped her chin on the floor.

Eric didn't notice. But then Eric never would. Ever the affable chap, life to him was a ball. He could take whatever you threw at him. If he didn't like it – no sweat – he'd just let it bounce off him. Take his tiff with Alex Ryman – his golfing buddy on Wednesday afternoons – their friendship had soon been back on course, no lasting handicap there. So I knew Lucy would have to be far below par before Eric would notice.

Not so Crystal. She had a canny instinct for knowing when things weren't quite right. So I wasn't surprised when she broached the subject with me.

'Thought I'd have a word with you first, Paul,' she said, 'rather than embarrassing Lucy.' She smoothed down the folds of her cream skirt, the gold bangles on her wrists tingling as she did so. It sent a similar wave of tingles down my spine. Maria ... Maria ... I once knew a girl called— Sorry. Getting confused. That was *West Side Story* not *The Sound of Music*. With a puzzled look, she straightened up and squared her shoulders, a no-nonsense stance adopted. 'I take it all's well between you and her? As I'm sure you're aware, I'm never that happy when personal relationships develop between staff. If it works, fine, but if it doesn't ... well....' She grimaced. 'It makes it uncomfortable for everyone concerned.'

I reassured her that we were getting along fine. Well, we were, really. Weren't we?

'And I know it's not my place to interfere, but whatever the problem is, I hope you're able to discuss it with her. We can't have her going round looking so glum. It's bad for morale and not good for the clients to see.'

I couldn't disagree with that. But getting Lucy to talk about it? I had tried. It was like trying to prise open a clam with a rubber fork. Besides, even if she did shell out her problem, I felt sure it wouldn't be palatable.

The next chance I had was the following Thursday. We both finished early that afternoon and it meant there was still time to snatch a few moments of sunshine on the patio back at Willow Wren. It was an almost identical scene to the previous Saturday. The loungers, a wasp or two, a few barbed comments and the tortoiseshell cat. Having failed to prise anything out of Lucy, I turned my attention to the local paper. Not that I was a particular fan of the *Westcott Gazette* but I did try to keep up with what was going on. And the paper did have its uses. The demise of the oak tree on the Green and the arrival of Cyril the squirrel at the hospital had made for good copy. And old editions made excellent liners for the cages.

It was as I opened the paper that I felt the swish of a tail against my elbow. There was a soft, intermittent purr, hesitant, uncertain. I raised my elbow and looked down to find the tortoiseshell cat staring up with those yellow eyes of hers questioning, her paws kneading the ground, first the left then the right as if marching on the spot. I looked across at Lucy. She was studying one of her nursing books. Holding the paper up as a screen between us, I patted my lap. 'OK, puss,' I whispered. She needed no further encouragement to nimbly spring up, turn one graceful circle on my knee and then curl into a ball, her purr at full throttle.

With the paper still held upright to conceal the cat, I became very well acquainted with what had been happening in the Westcott area during the last week. Within five minutes I'd learnt that Cicely Tingley had celebrated her 100th birthday; the Chawcombe and Ashton Afternoon Tea Group had released its autumn schedule and were meeting in Ashton village hall on Mondays at 3 p.m., at Westcott's Flower and Vegetable Show, Albert Cooper had won best of class for his leeks; and that the Christmas pantomime at the Pavilion was going to be *Aladdin* starring the famous TV actress, Francesca Cavendish – hmm. I wondered what genie would be stroking her lamp. A further five minutes ensured I was well acquainted with all the planning applications being considered by Westcott District Council and discovered I could lose up to 7 lb in two weeks at my local Rosemary Conley Class.

'Since when have you found the *Westcott Gazette* so interesting?' Lucy finally said. 'You're always telling me what a rag it is.'

I continued to hold the paper up in front of me, arms outstretched even though they were getting a bit tired by now. 'I think it's important to keep up with what's going on locally.' The cat chose that moment to wake up. She stood and arched her back, her tail like a mast, its tip quivering above the paper; it was instantly spotted by Lucy.

Clam or no clam, there was the unmistakable hiss of some valve opening as Lucy expressed her disapproval. It was enough to make the tortoiseshell cat shoot off my lap and disappear next door.

'Hope we've seen the back of her,' was Lucy's parting shot.

I found myself thinking what a pity. But heaven knows why. After all there were countless cats looking for homes. The noticeboard at Prospect House was testimony to that. It bristled with cards requesting homes for unwanted kittens. There was that ginger tom whose owners were emigrating. And that sleek, independent Siamese, Suki – her owners had just divorced. So why should I bother about some poor little scrap of a tortoiseshell?

The next day's long list of cat speys and castrations soon brought me to my senses. As each uterus and pair of testicles plopped into the kidney dish so did my gut feeling about taking on another cat. By the sixth castration they were well and truly emasculated. At least so I thought.

That lunchtime I decided on impulse to nip home. Although it meant a fifteen-minute drive over the Downs to Ashton, Lucy and I occasionally allowed ourselves the luxury of doing so as it meant a break from Prospect House. Lucy told me she had to stay.

'Mandy wanted to go into town this lunchtime. She asked me to cover for her. Couldn't very well say no, as she's the boss,' she added tersely. 'But it doesn't stop you going.' She gave a dismissive shrug of the shoulders.

For a moment I thought perhaps I should also stay. But to be honest I was getting fed up with her sullen moods and so felt no guilt as I headed back to Willow Wren without her. It was fate that I did so.

As I headed over the Downs I kept thinking of our relationship. It seemed to have hit a bit of a rocky patch. Which was stupid really as we had so much in common. I felt a bit of a wimp for not trying harder to find out what was unsettling Lucy so much. Yes, Beryl had told me about her and Mandy not getting on lately, but I hadn't noticed anything too untoward. True there was a bit of tension between them. But what was new?

Mandy ruled the roost. She was Fox by name and fox by nature. Smart with a streak of cunning which ensured that she managed to get her own way whenever possible and manipulated situations to ensure she was seen in the best light. Yes. Quite the little vixen. One that, if you ran it to earth, could turn on you with some savagery.

The main road from the Downs heading north skirted Ashton. You had to turn off down a slip road to reach the village. Never a problem to come off the road but certainly one to get on it. Especially first thing in the morning when trying to get out from the T-junction, a constant stream of commuter traffic heading south for Westcott making the wait at the junction a frustrating one. And dangerous. Oncoming cars to the left dipped out of sight before reaching the junction so that many a time you thought it was clear to shoot out only to have a car blasting its horn up your rear as you pulled away.

Seems something like that had happened now. As I slowed to turn off there were two cars parked to the side of the junction, a knot of people huddled between them. One was the cassocked figure of Revd

Matthews, crouched on the ground, his hands clasped together. Oh dear, surely he wasn't administering the last rites to someone. He looked up, caught sight of me, jumped to his feet and started to flail his arms above his head. I had no choice but to draw in behind them and stop.

'Ah, Mr Mitchell. How fortuitous of you to have arrived at this precise moment in time considering the gravity of the situation we have on our hands,' he said in a torrent of words, as I approached. 'There's been a most unfortunate accident. Most unfortunate. A dear little cat's been run over. Mrs Spencer here saw it happen.' He pointed to Joan who was kneeling by the cat, stroking its head.

'I was just on my way back to the post office,' she said, as I crouched down beside her. 'I think it's the little tortoiseshell that's been hanging around here this last week or so.'

She was right. It was the cat that only yesterday had been curled up, blissfully purring on my lap and who now lay sprawled on the side of the road, blood seeping from under her.

'Reckon she's a goner,' declared one of the bystanders.

Revd Matthews leapt forward, his cassock flapping vigorously as another car shot past in a whistle of wind. 'I think the cat's condition should be ascertained by someone who has the professional ability to carry out the necessary....' Further words were drowned by the roar of a juggernaut that came thundering over the brow of the hill. But the gist of what he had been saying was clear and I was allowed to examine the tortoiseshell cat without further comment.

There was blood coming from her mouth, her pupils were dilated, the eyes glazed and the breathing irregular. But at least she was still alive. She seemed a fighter. This was going to be a severe test for her.

The driver of the car which had hit her – a smart young man in suit and tie – offered to take the cat to the hospital. I thanked him, but said I'd take her back myself and phoned Prospect House to warn them I was coming in with an RTA. But the line was busy.

When I arrived, I was greeted by an agitated Beryl. 'Oh Paul, thank goodness you're back,' she said in a hoarse whisper, hand cupped characteristically over the side of her mouth. 'Crystal's had to make an emergency visit to Lady Derwent. She's asked if you'd cover her appointments until she gets back. Two have arrived early. They're in the waiting-room now.'

It was my turn to become agitated. I had the tortoiseshell cat in the back of the car. She really had to take priority. I charged down the corridor hollering for Lucy. It was Mandy who appeared first from the prep room, Lucy close behind her.

'What's the problem?' said Mandy, bustling forward.

'An RTA. A cat.' I looked over her shoulder at Lucy. 'It's that little tortoiseshell. She's on a blanket in the back of my car.'

'I'll get her,' said Lucy, pushing past both of us with alacrity.

By the time we'd got the cat in the prep room and a drip set up for her, two more of Crystal's clients had arrived. I could hear Beryl apologizing for the delay in being seen. The cat remained flat out, unconscious. The bleeding from the mouth was due to a broken tooth, nothing too serious. I quickly palpated her limbs. No breaks detected. But there was a grating noise from the pelvic area as I lifted her hindquarters. 'I'm going to have to get that X-rayed after I've seen Crystal's appointments,' I said, before dashing out.

When I returned half-an-hour later I found it had just been done.

'Seeing how busy you are, I thought it would save time,' said Mandy chirpily. 'I've taken a ventro-dorsal view of the pelvis and a lateral of the spine. Lucy's developing them now.'

For a moment I was dumbstruck. Surely Mandy had overstepped the mark here? After all, I hadn't given instructions as to what X-rays to take. Not that they would have been any different. Perhaps then I should be admiring her for taking the initiative?

Mandy went on, 'Crystal often lets me X-ray her cases when she's pushed for time.' She gave me one of her doe-eyed stares, brimming with defiance.

Maybe, I thought, but not without full instructions first. I was about to make a comment but decided it wiser not to as just then the darkroom door opened and Lucy emerged. 'The X-rays are ready,' she said quietly.

'Then bring them out please,' said Mandy. 'We're waiting to see them.'

I noticed the 'royal we'. It gave me an inkling of what was bugging Lucy. I could see Lucy bite her bottom lip as she turned back into the darkroom and re-emerge, holding two radiographs.

Mandy snatched them from her and clipped them up on the viewing screen. 'Hmm. Just as I suspected,' she said, studying them closely. 'Multiple fractures of the pelvis.'

'Er ... excuse me, Mandy, may I?' I stepped forward and started looking at the X-rays myself. The lateral view of the spine revealed no obvious damage to the spinal vertebrae though this didn't rule out the possibility of spinal trauma as nerves could still be crushed without the damage being seen on an X-ray. Did Mandy know that?

Seems she did, since she said, 'That doesn't mean to say there's no damage to the spinal cord.'

Grr. As to the pelvis, Mandy was right there too. There were multiple fractures. Another grr. Talk about nerves. This little madam was certainly beginning to get on mine.

Whatever. We ... sorry ... I had a cat with a paralysed back. The bystander's words came back to me – 'Reckon she's a goner.' For a moment I did wonder. Was I being unkind to keep her alive? Then I remembered Mrs Munroe's corgi. That had seemed a hopeless case with the X-ray showing a vertebra had dislocated upwards, crushing the spinal cord causing complete paralysis of the hindquarters. Yet Mrs Munroe had insisted on giving the dog a chance. And though it took over six weeks, he did manage to walk again.

Trouble was here the little tortoiseshell cat didn't have anyone to champion her cause. No owner to support her. No one but us to help nurse her through the difficult days and weeks ahead.

'Doesn't look too good,' said Mandy, still looking at the X-rays.

'I think we should give her a chance,' Lucy suddenly declared.

Mandy turned on her. 'She'll take a lot of nursing. There'll be no bladder control. So that will have to be emptied manually each day. And she's bound to get constipated. It could take weeks before we see any improvement.' From her tone it was clear she was far from enthusiastic about the idea.

'I still think it's worth a go,' said Lucy, her voice suddenly filling with determination. 'Even if you don't.'

Wow. That's my girl, I thought. You go for it.

Mandy whirled round on me, her cheeks flushed, eyes questioning.

Now, of course, I was in no doubt as to what to say. And I said it with glee. 'We'll try.'

Of course, the job of looking after the tortoiseshell cat was relegated to Lucy. No surprises there. But she didn't seem to mind – even though it was an onerous task and time-consuming.

I watched one such session. The cat's bladder manually expressed, the faecal boluses carefully manipulated out, the hindquarters washed down, dried and dusted with talcum powder. It was done with quiet efficiency. No sign of emotion. No sentiments expressed.

'Sweet little thing, isn't she?' I said, hoping to provoke some response. But no. Lucy just got on with the task without comment.

'No one's claimed her, you know.' Actually Lucy did know. I was just reminding her of the fact. Joan Spencer had put a card up in the post office and the vicar had mentioned her at the end of one of his sermons. Bless him. But nobody had come forward though several people reported they'd been visited by her for short periods. Never for long. No one it seems had come up to her expectations.

'Yet she's so friendly,' I persisted. 'Can't imagine she's a feral cat.' Still no response from Lucy.

Three days after the accident, the tortoiseshell cat was strong enough to lift herself up on her front legs. During my morning ward rounds, I'd tickle her whiskers and she'd respond by rubbing her head against my fingers, purring loudly.

By the end of the week she'd peed of her own accord. I caught Lucy recording the fact on the cat's clinical card.

'Why, that's marvellous,' I exclaimed

'It's a start,' she replied, her voice devoid of emotion.

Over the ensuing days, the reflexes in the cat's back legs returned. She twisted round to look when I pricked the skin of her rump. She began to flick her tail – until now it had been limp, without the slightest bit of movement.

'Great,' I enthused. 'She's on the mend.'

'But we're not out of the woods yet,' remarked Lucy, glancing down the ward to where Mandy was busying herself preparing medications, pretending not to listen in.

That glance said it all. Of course. How stupid not to have realized. This was a test case: Lucy was out to prove herself. Desperate to see the cat pull through. Willing it to happen, but didn't want to let her feelings be known. Hence the detached attitude, the apparent lack of interest. All a smoke screen.

And I'd deduced that all from one glance? Well, possibly not. Maybe I was being too clever. Reading too much into it.

When the tortoiseshell cat finally managed to stagger to her feet. I saw it happen and let out a hoot of joy. 'Yippee,' I cried. 'She's made it, Luce.'

The cat, trembling, was standing, her hindquarters leaning against the cage wall for support. But nevertheless standing. I was pleased for her and Lucy.

'So I see,' said Lucy, scribbling the details on the cat's card, impassive as ever.

When the cat started tottering a few steps, the inevitable question arose. Space was needed in the ward. The cat needed somewhere to convalesce. Now here was the acid test. Was the boil just about to be lanced?

'Well, how about it?' I asked Lucy.

'It's up to you. It's your cottage.'

'Nonsense. You're part and parcel of it.'

'That's just it, Paul. I don't feel that way. There or here. Especially here.' The 'here' of that particular moment was the prep room where Mandy had instructed Lucy to make up the next day's sets of instruments for surgery and get them autoclaved. The pressure in the autoclave was fast building. And so too were the feelings in Lucy to judge from her face which had gone very white, two red blotches appearing on each cheek. Tears glistened on her long eyelashes. 'I sometimes think I'm just taken for granted. A general dogsbody at the beck and call of everyone.' With a sob, Lucy made for the door. I stepped across and barred her way.

'Now listen, Luce. You've got it all wrong. There's no way you're just taken for granted. You're very much needed by me and by the hospital.' I gripped her shoulders and stared into her hazel eyes. 'But especially by me. You have to believe that, OK?'

A tear began to roll down her cheek.

I lifted a finger and gently wiped it away. 'And I'm not the only one that needs you,' I whispered. 'There's a certain little tortoiseshell cat whose life you've helped to save – despite the odds stacked against her.' And despite Mandy's misgivings I said to myself. 'That cat still needs you, you know. In just the same way I still need you.'

I pulled her to me and kissed the tears away and was just planting my lips firmly on hers when Eric bounced in.

'Whoops, sorry,' he said. 'Bit hot in here.' And bounced out.

But the deed had been done. The boil lanced. All the bad feelings had been drained out.

The tortoiseshell cat came home.

Lucy seemed happier now. She'd made her point. Had taken a stance against Mandy and won. Yet even so, I felt our relationship wasn't what it was. That initial spark had dimmed somewhat. I was still nuts about the girl but I felt my feelings weren't reciprocated quite so strongly.

'Perhaps I'm just imagining it,' I said, addressing the tortoiseshell cat as she sat looking out of the French windows.

It was another gem of a day. Trees had now turned to burnished gold and brown; crisp leaves danced in whorls on the patio.

Despite having three cats and Nelson in the cottage, the tortoiseshell had remained distant from them. She displayed an indifference that in a human would be considered sullenness. Perhaps the cat too was depressed, frustrated that she could only hobble about with a limp, her right hindleg withered; certainly she didn't move far – her favourite spot was by the French windows, gazing out. Perhaps she yearned to escape? Perhaps Lucy did as well, feeling mentally if not physically crippled? She was certainly sullen. No really, Paul ... you're just being fanciful. Letting your imagination run away with you.

Whatever, today the tortoiseshell cat was showing even more interest in the garden than ever. Maybe it was just those leaves swirling around out there, or perhaps she did want to escape.

To date I hadn't let her out. There hadn't seemed much point when she could hardly move. But maybe no harm could come from now letting her out onto the patio. Let it be a test run – or rather test hobble.

'Come on then, little one. We'll give it a try.' I opened one of the doors and she stiffly got to her feet and slowly limped onto the patio where she flopped down again in a pool of sunshine.

It was then I spotted the cat in the shrubbery. The broad head of a tom. A large black tom with saucer-shaped mint-green eyes. Eyes that were fixed intently on the tortoiseshell cat. After a few minutes he slipped from the bushes and padded up to her, his tail straight as a flag pole. He circled her, clearly puzzled as to why she didn't get up to greet this fine gentleman who was paying his respects. But he behaved with impeccable manners and backed off to sit a few feet away and give his whiskers a perfunctory wash.

Having seen the tortoiseshell cat's disdain of our three cats, I was surprised when she suddenly struggled to her feet and limped over to him slowly. Courteous to a fault, he stopped his ablutions and stood up. She drew nearer, their noses touched. A friendship was struck.

From that moment on, the little tortoiseshell improved mentally and physically. She showed much more interest in life. Whereas before, I had to go and find her, entice her to eat, she now walked stiffly into the kitchen, rubbed herself against my legs and demanded her breakfast with a loud purr. She began to move about more easily, always eager to be let out, weather permitting, and was soon able to negotiate the steps from the patio onto the lawn.

The black cat continued to visit, his broad beaming face suddenly appearing in the lower right-hand pane of the French windows where the little tortoiseshell began to wait for him, eager for his companionship.

By now, she'd gained as much use of her hind legs as she was likely to, the wasted muscles of her right leg the only sign of permanent damage. It meant she couldn't jump onto my lap like she used to when she first visited Willow Wren, but now, even if I lifted her up, she never stayed long. She spent most of her time by the French windows as if biding her time until she was fit enough to leave us altogether. So the day she vanished came as no real surprise.

'Just hope she's OK,' I said to Lucy, staring out at the blanket of soggy leaves which now covered the patio and lawn.

'Don't fret,' replied Lucy. 'She's an independent sort. She wasn't going to stay forever.' I was waiting for her to add 'Like me' for there were echoes of Lucy in that cat's character. I just prayed that she wouldn't get it into her head to leave me as well.

The next day I did begin to fret. The weather had turned atrocious. Heavy, black clouds scudded across a dismal lowering grey sky. Rain lashed down, pelting against the windows. Surely the little tortoiseshell would have been happier indoors, stretched out in front of the fire, enjoying the warmth, enjoying the regular meals – even if she didn't have the black cat for company.

The black cat. It suddenly struck me. He hadn't been seen for the last few days ever since the tortoiseshell had gone missing. Yes. That black tom. I pictured him at the French window. Then another image came to mind. Another black cat framed in a pane of glass. The cat in Major Fitzherbert's greenhouse. Leo – or rather Cuddles as he was now called. Could he be one and the same cat?

I was on the phone immediately.

'Hello, Major Fitzherbert here.' The familiar voice barked down the line.

'Er … sorry to trouble you on a Sunday, Major. It's Mr Mitchell here.'

'Mitchell?'

'The vet.' I took a deep breath and started to explain. 'So I'm wondering whether she's turned up at your place,' I concluded.

There was a pause followed by a deep-throated chuckle. 'Well, young sir, I reckon she has. A slip of a thing has been keeping Cuddles company here these last couple of days. The two of them are snoozing in front of the fire this very minute. She fits your description so I guess she must be yours.'

The mention of 'yours' didn't ring true somehow. She'd never really been mine. We hadn't bonded together. I found myself explaining this to the major and added, 'She's what you might call an independent sort and has never been at home here.'

The major gave another throaty chuckle. 'Just the sort of cat I admire. Still, she seems to have shacked up with Cuddles for the time being. What say we give them a chance together? Would you mind?'

Did I mind? Part of me said 'Yes, I did' the other told me I was being selfish, too possessive, I should let her go. The latter won.

I couldn't help thinking the same about Lucy. As I climbed into bed that night and snuggled down next to her, it was still on my mind. Was I being too possessive about her as well? Too self-centred? Only thinking of my welfare. Not hers. Unwilling to let her go should she chose to do so.

It was Lucy who spoke first. 'Paul, I've been thinking....'

I felt a knot tighten in my stomach.

'That cat....'

'What about her?'

'You knew she'd never settle. That she'd never be yours.'

'Well, yes, I did,' I admitted. 'How did you know?'

'Think about it.'

I did and eased myself closer.

'All the time you spent pulling her through the accident, never once did you think of giving her a name. That surely proves something. That she didn't really belong. That she wasn't yours.'

I nuzzled Lucy's neck, felt her soft hair fall across my cheek, felt her warmth, breathed in her scent. She was right. The cat had always been just that: the little tortoiseshell cat. Never named. Never mine. 'But you've got a name, Luce,' I whispered. 'And I'd like you to be mine, all mine, and never leave me,' I added, enfolding her in my arms.

Chapter 13

'You're getting quite a reputation,' remarked Mandy, as I tied off the last stitch, the bitch spey completed.

'Really?' I replied. This sounded interesting. Perhaps Crystal had noticed I was becoming a dab hand at operating. All these speys and castrates making me sharp with the knife. Why, I could now winkle out an ovary in the shake of a lamb's tail. Baa. So what? It wasn't exactly cutting-edge stuff – not in the sense of complicated surgery. That still tended to fall into Crystal's hands. No slice of it came my way.

Mandy made a fuss of dabbing the minute trickle of blood that oozed from one corner of the wound before whipping off the spey cloths and disconnecting the endotrachael tube from the anaesthetic machine in her customary efficient manner.

'Come on then,' I urged, pulling off my surgical gloves, sweat showering out of them. 'What's this about a reputation.'

Mandy sprinkled some antibiotic powder alone the line of the wound and covered it with a thin strip of cotton wool before looking up. 'Seems you've become our bird expert.'

Oh. So that was it, was it? Paul Mitchell the man you had to see if your Joey needed his bill trimmed or the canary her claws cut. Some reputation. I blamed it on Beryl. She was the one who kept pushing the birds onto me and then only because Eric and Crystal didn't want to deal with them. The trend had started with Miss McEwan's mynah and, as the summer flew past, so did the number of feathered patients that winged their way through my surgery.

Later that day I was able to add one more to my ever-increasing flock.

'Another budgie, is it, Beryl?' I asked.

'Ooh no. I've booked you in something much, much better than that,' she said, crowing with glee and swinging back and forth on her stool to such an extent that I thought she'd become airborne any moment. 'Mrs Smethurst's got a cockatoo.'

And what a moth-eaten specimen Liza turned out to be.

'Yes. I'm afraid she is a bit of a mess,' apologized Mrs Smethurst, sliding the large parrot cage on to the consulting table.

'Almost ready for the oven,' I joked unwisely, as the almost naked cockatoo waddled up and down her perch.

'Everyone cracks that one,' sighed Mrs Smethurst, 'but it's beyond a joke. Liza simply won't stop pulling her feathers out. We're getting quite desperate.' Her pert nose gave a rabbit-like twitch.

The cockatoo raised her crest and bobbed her head at me. That head was still quite appealing with its white cheeks and crest feathers dusted with yellow. But the only other feathers remaining were the half-chewed ones on her wings and tail. In between, nothing. Not a single feather to cover her nakedness. Just a sea of skin – grey, pimply and utterly repulsive.

'So how long has she been feather plucking?' I asked.

'I guess it must be about three months now. Ever since my sister went to Australia. Liza was hers really.'

'And how long had she owned her?'

There was another rabbit twitch of the nose. 'Must have been at least four years. More likely five.'

'And no problems during that time?'

'None whatsoever. My sister adored the bird. They were seldom out of each other's sight.'

'I'd say that's the most likely reason then. A psychosomatic disorder.'

Mrs Smethurst's forehead furrowed in confusion.

I explained. 'Liza's missing your sister. She needs some distractions.'

She's not the only one I thought, averting my eyes from Mrs Smethurst's denim shirt unbuttoned to her cleavage.

I took a deep breath and expanded on my plan of action.

Over the ensuing weeks, Mrs Smethurst inundated Liza with plastic ducks and budgies. All fell easy prey to her beak. Lengths of chain were shortened by the hour, their links dextrously unpicked. A toy bell barely managed a tinkle before it cracked up.

'Don't know about the bell, but I could wring her neck,' complained

Mrs Smethurst, as Liza continued to chew her feather stumps.

'Try a mirror,' I suggested.

One was placed next to Liza's cage. Useless. She just watched herself plucking, occasionally strutting up to the mirror to peer at her reflection as if to see what remaining feathers she could yank out.

'Change the food and water hoppers around every day.'

Liza found herself climbing up to reach her peanuts; climbing down for some fruit; up again for a drink. No good.

'Reposition her perches.'

They were raised, lowered, sloped to the right, sloped to the left. Still she plucked.

'Add some more.'

Extra were crammed in: different woods, smaller twigs, bigger branches. Her cage became like the Forest of Arden. It might have been *As She Liked It* for Liza, with her in the centre of the glade merrily plucking, not a lyre, but the vestiges of her plumage. But if I could have struck a cord, it would have been one thrown over a bough of a Greenwood tree while I hummed a merry note as it was tied round Liza's throat. The bird was driving me nuts.

'Try putting her cage in a different place every day.'

'Have done. Even the bathroom. But those beady eyes staring at me. So embarrassing. Besides which she started imitating the cistern.' Mrs Smethurst's cheeks flushed. 'But it hasn't done the slightest bit of good as you can see.'

Indeed I could see. No good at all.

The facts were before me. Bare facts. Liza waddled across her perch, raised the three remaining feathers on her crest and puffed out her chest in all its naked glory.

'I'm afraid we'll have to resort to an Elizabethan collar,' I sighed. 'She won't like it though.'

'No, she won't,' echoed Lucy, as I showed her how to cut out a circle of plastic from some old X-ray film before she helped me loop it round Liza's neck to form a cone. 'See?'

The cockatoo craned her neck out and gave an indignant screech.

'She'll quieten down.' I bundled Liza back into her cage. She rolled over and lay momentarily on her back, silent, her chest heaving, the pimply skin pulsating in time to her heart, her head out-of-sight in the cone. Suddenly, with a thrash of her legs, she flipped over, doing a complete somersault to land precisely in the same position. With scarcely a pause, she did it again. And again.

Lucy began to giggle. 'She's flipped her lid,' she said.

'Shush … it's no laughing matter,' I said. But I could feel a bubble of laughter welling up in my throat.

Liza spun over three times, hit the metal bars of the cage, gripped, and blindly climbed her way up, the cone crashing wildly from side to side, slamming against food hoppers and bars alike. She reached the top and stopped, her head out of sight, the cone pressed up against the roof of the cage. She suddenly relaxed her grip and shot rapidly down the bars.

By now Lucy was convulsed with giggles, her eyes streaming.

'Shh … shh,' I implored, 'Mrs Smethurst might hear you.' But the bubble of laughter in my throat was about to burst out. I rammed my knuckles into my mouth as I tried to stop it.

Meanwhile, Liza had clawed her way back up and dropped down again. Only to zoom back up and spiral down yet again. She was like an animated yo-yo. Up down. Up down.

Ha … Ha … Ha. Out poured the laughter. *Hee. Hee … Hee. Oh dear God, pleasssse.* But no. It was uncontrollable. I was as helpless as a kitten. Splitting my sides. Lucy, too, was squirming and writhing, an explosion of giggles. We hopped and skipped round the prep room, bent over, arms wrapped tightly round our chests. *Ha … Ha … Ha … Hee … Hee … Hee.* Impossible to stop. Oh deary me. What a laugh. What a scream.

'What the hell's going on?'

The voice was sharp and crystal clear. Crystal Sharpe's to be precise. The door had been thrown open and she was standing there looking at us. Unlike us, she was not amused. Far from it.

I reeled to a halt.

'S … s … sorry, Crystal,' I spluttered. 'It's just that….' My voice rose to squeak. 'It's just that….' My voice rose even higher. *Tee … hee …hee.* I caught sight of Liza now standing on her head, the cone acting as a base, her naked legs pedalling the air above her. It was all too much. Another wave of giggles spilled out. *Tee … hee … hee.*

'It's not funny,' snapped Crystal, marching over to the cage where she reached in and turned Liza the right way up. 'There's a client up in reception wondering what all the commotion is about. I take it this is her bird?'

I nodded, my sides aching, my eyes feeling swollen and bleary.

'Well, you'd better go and explain yourself,' continued Crystal.

With that, she spun on her heels and stormed out. Whoops. There goes my Julie Andrews.

Mrs Smethurst was dubious when she saw her collared cockatoo. 'Are you sure she's not going to harm herself?' she queried.

'No, really. I think she'll get used to it quite soon,' I replied with more conviction than I felt. 'But if there are any problems please don't hesitate to get in contact.'

She did, five hours later, when I'd just got into bed.

Mandy was on night duty and phoned to say Mrs Smethurst thought Liza was dying.

My feet hit the floor with a thud.

'Not that damned parrot again?' mumbled Lucy, next to me.

'Cockatoo,' I corrected, hopping around as I struggled into my jeans. 'Mrs Smethurst thinks she's snuffing it.'

'Plucked herself to death, shouldn't wonder,' yawned Lucy, snuggling back down under the duvet.

By the time I'd driven to Prospect House, Mandy had let Mrs Smethurst in and the cage was on the consulting table.

'So much for your collar,' said Mrs Smethurst. 'It's done for Liza.'

I peered into the cage. Liza was lying prostrate on the floor, motionless, her claws tucked into the neck of the cone, her chest heaving in small, spasmodic jerks. I unbolted the cage door and dragged the bird out. She lay in the palm of my hand without a struggle, not a murmur, not a squawk. It really seemed she was on her last legs.

'Legs,' I exclaimed.

Mrs Smethurst frowned, her rabbit-nose twitched.

'Liza's legs,' I went on. 'Look.' I got hold of one and tugged. It wouldn't budge. 'That's why she's so still. She's stuck. See?' I showed Mrs Smethurst how Liza's sharp claws had pierced the X-ray film and had made her immobile. When I'd extracted her claws, she began to thrash around once more.

'I'm sorry, but I can't go through all that again,' protested Mrs Smethurst.

'No, of course not,' I agreed and snipped through the knots and removed the collar.

Liza strutted up and down her perch triumphantly. Then she stopped, twisted her head over her back, yanked out a broken tail feather and held it in her claws, waving it to and fro like a banner at a victory parade.

Mrs Smethurst sighed. 'She really is the limit. I don't how much longer I can put up with her.'

It turned out to be a month. One blustery October day I was presented with the moth-eaten bird and asked if I could find a new home for her.

'It's a long story,' said Mrs Smethurst, taking a deep breath, her bosoms expanding against her cashmere sweater.

'No hurry,' I murmured, my eyes drawn to the sweater like two flies to a pear. 'There's plenty of time.'

Mrs Smethurst took another nice, deep breath and began. It seems she had started to let Liza out of her cage each day in the hope it would be an extra distraction for her. Yesterday evening, she had walked in, her hair in curlers. Liza, perhaps thinking the curlers were some sort of new toy, flew across and landed on her head. There followed, by all accounts, an agonizing tussle as Liza got caught up in a curler, started flapping and scrabbling, her claws digging into the poor woman's scalp.

Here Mrs Smethurst's face contorted at the memory. She paused and drew a hand over her sweater. 'Sorry, if you could just bear with me a moment,' she said, with a little quiver.

'No problem,' I replied, with a bigger quiver.

Once more composed, she continued. She had staggered about, both she and Liza screaming, getting in an absolute tizz. Her husband had rushed to the rescue with a towel, smothering the bird and his wife's head. He had finally managed to prise Liza off along with a clump of hair.

'Can you imagine how it felt?' declared Mrs Smethurst, taking another deep breath.

Oh yes ... yes ... yes. Indeed I could.

The bird had to go, concluded Mrs Smethurst. Would I take her? Oh yes ... yes ... yes. Indeed I would.

'You did what?' screeched Lucy that evening.

Before I could explain, there was a loud squawk from the hall. Liza, pleased to hear a kindred spirit had screeched in reply.

We soon learnt what that screech meant. Don't dare leave me. If you do, I'll screech the house down until you return. It was the sort of screech that went right through the wall; the sort that screeched through the ceiling and screeched through your cranium, setting your nerves on edge like nails raking down a blackboard. Even Joan and George next door heard it and phoned to enquire whether all was well and was it some sort of sick chicken that we were treating.

Liza didn't squawk so much if let out; so for the sake of our eardrums she was allowed more and more freedom.

Having given the room the once-over to make sure Nelson or Queenie and her friends weren't around to upset her, she'd fix her beady eye on me, give a 'Here I come' squawk and soar across to land on the back of the settee. Here, she'd bob up and down, her three remaining crest feathers raised, her naked neck stretched out. Her crop often bulged, the white gleam of lumps of peanut showing through the thin grey skin like a nodular abscess about to burst.

With scarcely any plumage left to savage, she decided to have a go at the three remaining crest feathers on the top of her head. To achieve this required considerable dexterity. She would balance on one leg, raise the other foot and tilt her head down to grab a crest feather in her claws. Then she'd tug and tug, pulling her head lower and lower as she tried to wrench the feather out. More often than not, she'd yank so hard that she'd lose her balance and topple forward, cartwheeling down the side of the settee only to scramble back up with an indignant squawk and try again.

'She needs more distractions,' stated Lucy.

'I've been through all that with Mrs Smethurst,' I said. 'Short of another bird as a companion. Hey ... maybe that's the answer.'

'Don't even think about it,' warned Lucy.

I shrugged. 'Shouldn't worry. It's highly unlikely as cockatoos don't come cheap.'

'No they come bloody squawking,' complained Lucy, stuffing her fingers in her ears as Liza let rip again – this time alarmed by the sight of a lion stalking across the TV screen.

It was barely a week later when Major flew into our lives. A client from another practice heard I was a 'bird man' and phoned to ask if I'd be interested in taking on her cockatoo. I went round to see the bird.

'Does Major ... er ... squawk?' I asked, standing in front of the cage. He had been suspiciously quiet since my arrival.

'Very rarely,' said the lady and went on to explain that Major had been her son's, but now that he'd left home there was no one to devote time to the bird.

'Doesn't feather pluck, I see.' Major had a full compliment of smart white feathers and a fine sweep of a yellow tipped crest.

'No, he's got no vices,' said the lady vaguely. 'Nothing to speak of that is.'

Well, there was a vice. A vice not mentioned. A vice only discovered when I got Major home.

We were in the kitchen when a commotion erupted from the sitting-room. It sounded like someone beating the hell out of a tin kettle.

'What on earth's that racket?' said Lucy, almost dropping the eggs she'd been taking out of the fridge. I ran in to investigate.

For once, Liza was actually quiet, watching Major, her two remaining crest feathers raised in bewilderment. He, on the other hand was creating the noise, ramming his beak into his food hopper, beating it against the sides like some demented pop group's drummer.

'Perhaps that's why he's called Major,' said Lucy, when she came through.

'I don't follow.'

'Drum major,' she explained, as the cockatoo beat another tattoo in his hopper, scattering sunflower seed in all directions.

But Major hadn't finished yet. He looked up as if to make sure we were watching and then launched himself forward from his perch while still hanging on. The momentum in his dive allowed him to flip under the perch and haul himself back up the other side using his beak. He was like a Catherine wheel. A spinning blur of white. A real comic turn. Quite amazing.

It was a trick that subsequently never failed to make us smile especially on those occasions when it didn't quite come off and he was left swinging backwards and forwards, clinging to his perch upside down.

Liza chose to ignore this new joker and after that initial silence returned to her daily torrent of screeches directed solely at us.

Still, I put their cages side by side for a week and then decided to put the birds together. But in a new cage.

'Why a new one?' queried Lucy.

'Bit of psychology,' I explained. 'Meeting on new territory should help to lessen any aggression between them. There, look at that.'

Having been put in with Major, Liza had now run up to him, her remaining crest feather raised, her beak giving a friendly click click. 'They're making friends already.'

But Major wasn't having any of it. He huddled up against the side of the cage, his strident hiss making it clear he had no wish for flirtations from his Antipodean sister, already undressed, flaunting her naked flesh at him.

That night both birds roosted at opposite ends of the perch. We were woken at 5 a.m. by our own dawn chorus of screeches echoing up from the sitting-room.

'Now what?' moaned Lucy, burying her head under the pillow while her heel, planted firmly in the small of my back, ensured I was ejected to investigate.

Liza ran along the perch to give me a bob, her right wing dripping blood. Huddled at the other end, sat Major, the picture of innocence, except his beak was smeared with red.

The wound wasn't serious – a nick in the skin – so I decided to risk leaving the birds together. Foolish move. Another commotion in the early hours of the following morning, combined with Lucy's heel in my back again, forced me to change my mind. Liza was getting beaten up and my back was getting sore. The birds were separated.

From that moment on, they totally ignored each other. We would come into the room and they would each vie for our attention, screeches from Liza, hopper bashing and perch somersaults from Major. Each seemed to spur the other on to new heights of frenzy.

Lucy and I were finally driven to distraction when both birds added the other's repertoire to its own so that we ended up with two bobbing, somersaulting, hopper-bashing, screeching cockatoos. Major, having the more powerful lungs left us feeling as if Big Ben had been striking on our mantelpiece – we were totally tolled off and wrung out. All too much.

In desperation, I phoned a local garden centre that I knew had an aviary in its greenhouse section – designed to give a tropical ambience to the purchase of trays of pansies and petunias. The owner was more than willing to take on two cockatoos.

'For free you say?'

For free he was assured.

'What's wrong with them then?'

'Well they do screech a bit.'

'That's not a problem.'

'And one of them is a bit bald.'

'Bald? How bald?'

How could I describe Liza's condition other than as oven-ready? There was no way I could cover it – or her – up.

So Major went and Liza stayed. She seemed delighted at the arrangement. After all, she now had our undivided attention once more; and she could tweak out any new feathers that tried to grow through to her heart's content without interruption. We gave up hope of ever getting her to stop.

I wasn't too sure when the idea of the party was first muted. It was a bit like a sea of whispers. I overheard Mandy and Lucy discussing something down in the ward but they abruptly stopped conferring as soon as I walked in. Both looked guilty. So I knew something was afoot. But at least they were now talking to each other. It was as if the incident with the little tortoiseshell cat had been a watershed. Since then Lucy had been in a much better frame of mind, helped by a more co-operative Mandy who now tended to share her responsibilities with Lucy rather than treat her as the general dogs-body. She even permitted Lucy to take charge of the anaesthetic machine during a few routine operations. Closely supervised, of course. But, nevertheless, it proved there had been a significant shift in their relationship as the anaesthetic machine was usually jealously guarded by Mandy – very much her baby – not to be tampered with.

It was Beryl who let it slip. She had just finished smoking her coffee-break cigarette – having battled to puff the smoke out through a half-open back door while struggling with the door to stop the wind blowing it back in. Someone needed to tell her that her raven hair normally heavily lacquered to her head had sprouted wings and looked as if it was about to take off. But not me. No way.

'I don't know what to wear,' she said suddenly, giving me the eye as if I was about to inspire her. 'Fancy-dress parties aren't my sort of thing.'

'Party? What's this about a party?'

'You don't know?' She saw my quizzical look. 'No you don't, obviously. You'd better ask Lucy.' With that she quickly shimmied back up to reception.

'It's Mandy's idea,' said Lucy, when eventually I tracked her down in the dispensary making up a prescription – another job that Mandy now let her do unsupervised. 'She fancies having a bit of a knees-up.'

I shrugged. 'But where's she going to have it? I hardly think

Crystal and Eric would let her hold a party up in the flat. It would disturb all the in-patients. Let alone the neighbours.'

A block of flats had been built in the grounds sold off from Prospect House. People were forever complaining about the noise of dogs and cats. But, as Crystal said, we were there first. When the people bought those flats they knew exactly what they were letting themselves in for. But nevertheless, Crystal did her best to keep things on an even keel. A party in the flat would be rocking the boat too much.

'The flat's too small anyway,' said Lucy.

'Exactly.'

I saw her looking at me in a funny way. I knew Lucy well enough by now to know that look. It didn't bode well. A niggle of worry began to worm through me.

'Lucy, you're not suggesting—'

'Willow Wren would be perfect. It's certainly big enough.'

'Crystal wouldn't allow it.' I saw that look flash back into her eyes. 'Lucy! You haven't—'

'She said it was fine by her but to ask you. She and Eric are looking forward to coming.'

Hmm. Seems it was a done deal. I could hardly turn round and veto it without appearing to be a complete party pooper.

'And what's this about it being fancy-dress?'

'Mandy's idea. Thought fancy-dress would be a bit of fun. What were you wearing when the ship went down?'

It was enough to make my heart sink let alone a ship. I had visions of Willow Wren ending up a wreck.

In the event, it all went quite smoothly. And most people made an effort to dress up. With her wings of black hair I thought Beryl could have come as a crow's nest. But she turned up in her standard black trousers and top purporting to be the ship's cat. With her long claw-like nails and whiskery face she quite looked the part. Eric came as a stoker. He wore a dirty vest hanging out of grubby trousers, his face smeared with coal dust.

'Doesn't look much different to normal,' Beryl whispered to me, hand cupped to the side of her mouth. Catty ... catty ... she was playing her part well.

Crystal cruised through the crowd, very debonair as the ship's captain in crisp white uniform and gold braid on those lovely shaped shoulders of hers. Mmm. She could grab my bulwarks any time.

Lucy hummed and hahed for days beforehand, wondering what to wear. In the end, she decided on a long, white nightgown and powdered her face and arms with flour.

'What are you supposed to be?' I queried unwisely, as she thumped down the stairs, resembling a rolled out slab of pastry.

'A ship's ghost of course.'

She was thoroughly miffed when Mandy materialized in similar mode though, with her dumpy figure and naturally pallid complexion, Mandy looked the more frightful of the two.

And me? Well I plumped for Long John Silver. I had some baggy breeches, large buckled belt, a black, leather waistcoat and eye-patch. I stopped short of doing the one-legged bit in case I got leg-less.

'What about having Liza on your shoulder,' joked Lucy. 'I know she's not an Amazon Green but she'd do.'

The idea didn't appeal. I had visions of Liza being frightened by the crowd and flying around, panic stricken, landing, claws outstretched, in someone's hair à la Mrs Smethurst. Instead I visited the theatrical outfitters in Westcott.

'I'm afraid the best parrots are doing the rounds in rehearsals for *Treasure Island*,' apologized the assistant. 'This is all we have left.'

I viewed the two stuffed birds on offer. The African Grey shed a cloud of feathers as soon as I picked it up. Not a pretty Polly.

'How about the Amazon Green, then,' said the assistant, holding up the other bird.

By the looks of it, the parrot hadn't stood up too well to the ravages of countless pantomimes. Its emerald plumage was dull and dusty with a crumpled appearance accentuated by a wodge of flock sticking out between its legs and an eye dangling by a thread. But better the bird in hand than the one on the counter so I hired it.

With the party in full swing, I paraded around with the Amazon Green wired to the shoulder of my jacket. Liza squawked with jealousy when she saw it but was soon overwhelmed by the attention given her by the party-goers. She was inundated with titbits. The following morning I was to discover her cage floor littered with crisps, cocktail sticks with bits of pineapple still skewered to them, Twiglets, sausage rolls and, smeared to the bars, dollops of pâté.

Mandy floated over to me high on vodka and lime.

'Who's a pretty boy,' she said, her unfocused eyes staring up. Now was she referring to me, or the parrot on my shoulder? I assumed me as I didn't have an eye dangling out of its socket on a thin twist of wire. But it was to the bird she was giving the eye – her eye – as in the next second she reached up and yanked a bunch of feathers out of its tail.

'Mandy, what on earth…?'

But she'd gone, vanished in a swirl of sheets, the feathers doing likewise as they floated to the floor. Cursing, I craned my neck round to peer at the mutilated parrot only to discover someone had smeared cottage cheese down my jacket in imitation of bird droppings. How foul.

Then Liza was let out. The first I knew of it was when she landed on my shoulder with a friendly squawk, bobbed her tail and produced her own version of cottage cheese down my back.

Mandy hovered into view again, even more high-spirited. 'Wooo …wooo,' she said, raising her hands in the air, fingers fluttering. 'I'm a ship's ghost. Wooo … wooo.' She moved closer. 'Wooo … wooo.' If she was trying to scare me it didn't work. But it certainly frightened Liza.

With a shrill screech she lashed out at the fluttering fingers.

'Wooo … ouch … you little sod.' The fingers were snatched away, one dripping blood.

The next morning, with hammers in my head, I surveyed the mortal remains of the Amazon Green. It was tail-less, exposing a strand of rusty wire; the dangling eye had been lost revealing a white socket; the other eye was now loose and hanging out at an odd angle as if the bird was trying to study its toes; and its lower mandible had become dislocated and so twisted that the parrot appeared to be sneering at me. Worse still, more stuffing had worked loose so that the bird looked as if it were trying to give birth to an eiderdown.

'I can't possibly take it back in this state,' I moaned.

'Well, you're a vet. Stitch it up,' said Lucy less than sympathetic.

I took the parrot into work and attempted to operate on it, suturing with some nylon. But my trembling hands weren't up to it. The more I bundled the stuffing back and stitched across it, the more distorted the bird became. Its head swelled up and curled over like a dying duck while its back developed a hump worthy of Notre-Dame's bellringer. All resemblance to a parrot was lost.

Back home, I phoned the theatrical outfitters and explained the situation. The assistant was most sympathetic.

'It was on its last legs anyway,' he said. 'So I doubt if it would have survived another panto season.' He must have heard Liza squawking in the background as he suddenly added, 'Have you got a live one there?'

'Yes. A cockatoo.'

'Well, let us know if ever she snuffs it. We pay a good price.'

I didn't elaborate on Liza's condition. She'd never make a mounted specimen. But at least from that moment on, whenever her squawking provoked me to yell at her, it gave new meaning to the phrase 'Get stuffed', since I now knew where it could be done.

'So what are you going to do with it?' asked Lucy, looking at the disfigured Amazon Green. 'Throw it away?'

That had been my intention.

'Why not let Liza have it?' she continued. 'After all, it can't do her any harm. It's not as if it can peck her back.'

Liza stared suspiciously as the Amazon Green, wired to a broom handle, was propped up against her cage. But friendly as ever, she waddled up to the bars, raised her one remaining crest feather, and gave a little cluck. The lack of response clearly puzzled her. She gave another cluck – this time it was a little more strident. Still no reaction. Cautiously she pushed her beak between the bars and tweaked one of its feathers. The parrot rocked on his handle. Liza scuttled back down her perch.

As the parrot slowly came to a halt, Liza advanced again, clearly fascinated despite the creature's very un-parrot-like shape. She cooed and clucked at it: she snuggled up against the bars; she reached through and nibbled another of its feathers. Then with a frustrated screech, she yanked. Her head bobbed up, the feather dangling from her beak. She snatched it into her claws, stared down at it with one coal-black eye, ran her tongue over it, and then proceeded to mash it into a pulp before dropping it to the floor. Then, with scarcely a pause, she stretched through the bars and tweaked out another one.

Liza now had a friend unable to stop her advances. She spent hours preening it, gradually stripping it of its plumage while, untouched, hers began to grow through.

However, much to our disappointment, she still demanded attention from us. So the screeching never stopped. It began to wear us down.

I took to walking round with wax plugs wedged in my ears. Lucy wore ear muffs. But when Joan popped round and I couldn't understand a word she was saying, I realized something more constructive had to be done.

I tried the garden centre again but their aviary was now full. The theatrical outfitters began to feature more and more in my thoughts. Liza, resplendent now in her new white plumage, would be a taxidermist's delight.

'Don't be so cruel,' reprimanded Lucy. 'Liza just needs human company all the time. Someone who's potty about birds.'

'And deaf,' I shouted

'Try asking Beryl,' mouthed Lucy, ramming her ear muffs back down again as Liza started to join in the conversation.

'Let me think,' said Beryl, when I broached the subject with her over a cigarette at the back door. 'There's the vicar over at Chawcombe.'

'Not the one whose dog I gave first prize to at the fête?'

'Revd Venables. Yes. He and his wife are potty about parrots. They've got four of their own. Surprised they haven't been in to see you yet.'

I wasn't. Not after that débâcle last August.

'Well, what are you waiting for?' queried Lucy, when I told her of the Venables' love of parrots.

'It doesn't seem fair to burden someone else with Liza's screeching.'

'Oh for heaven's sake, don't be so soft. You say they've got four parrots already so I doubt if an extra squawk here or there will make any difference. Go on, give them a ring.'

'But really, I'd hate any comebacks.'

'Ring them.'

It was Liza who jolted me into action. She decided we'd done enough squawking of our own and joined in. It was a particularly piercing screech. How such little vocal cords could produce that intensity of noise I couldn't imagine. She must have puffed up her little lungs to their maximum capacity and let rip with all the power she could muster since the sound that vibrated through her larynx was like an express train's whistle as it thundered out of a tunnel. I flinched despite my ear plugs.

'Right, That's it. I've had enough,' I roared, storming out to snatch up the phone while prising out a plug.

*

As it turned out, the Venables were only too pleased to have Liza. I made the excuse she needed constant company.

'My dear, don't you worry,' gushed Mrs Venables, as Liza was installed in their drawing-room. 'She'll get all the company she needs. And I can't tell you how delighted we are to have a cockatoo. She's an absolute poppet. Just look at that beautiful plumage of hers.'

'Yes, she is pretty,' I admitted. 'But she is prone to the odd squawk.'

'My good man, don't you worry about that,' said Revd Venables with a beaming smile. It seemed he'd put the summer fête behind him. Either that or the fact he was getting a parrot for free was making him more solicitous. 'We have to put up with a lot of chatter from the others.' He turned and waved at the rest of his flock.

Balanced on their own occasional tables, were four large, stainless-steel parrot cages. Eight beady eyes stared intently out from them. Two pairs of African Greys. Two pairs of Amazon Greens.

'And quite the little congregation they are too, bless their hearts.' The vicar tilted his head to one side – why do vicars do that? – and added, 'I must confess that I read my sermons out to them.'

'That soon shuts them up,' said his wife.

'Thank you, my dear.' The vicar's head snapped back up and his lips tightened like a piece of string. The parrots remained silent. Even Liza was cowed.

I hurried from the vicarage, offering up thanks for my salvation and just prayed there'd be no repercussions.

When I next saw the vicar it was in Westcott's pet shop where he was buying a sack of parrot mix. I thought he looked a little weary. A little haggard. His cheeks were sallow and there were dark circles under his eyes. Perhaps he'd been partaking in too many late night masses?

'Liza's fine,' he replied to my enquiry. 'Such a sweet creature. We think the world of her. Only....' He hesitated. 'Well, she is rather vociferous. So much noise from such a little bird. Tends to break the concentration ... you know, when working on the next sermon.' The corner of his mouth twitched. A tic beat above his eye. 'But then you did warn us.' A tired smile flickered across his face and his hands trembled as he picked up the parrot mix. 'Still we do try letting her out as much as possible. In fact, she was on my shoulder this morning while I prepared tomorrow's lesson. At least it kept her quiet and enabled me to get on with my business.'

And to judge from what I saw, it had allowed Liza to get on with hers. As the vicar turned to leave the shop, I could see dollops of white splattered down the back of his cassock. But that was Liza for you. Life with her always did mean business.

Chapter 14

Although it wasn't yet November the fifth, Crystal burst in one morning all flash and sparkle – fizzing with such energy it would have put a Catherine wheel to shame. I on the other hand was more akin to a damp squid, the reason for my lack of spark the routine ops listed in the day-book awaiting my attention.

'Morning, Paul,' she said brightly, and flashed me one of her smiles. A smile that usually got my ticker racing. But not today – my heart wasn't in it. 'What glorious weather,' she added, striding energetically across to the window to gaze out, rubbing her dainty hands together.

Yes, I thought. It certainly is. A crisp morning with a cool blue sky. The sort of day to get out-of-doors if one possibly could. And Crystal certainly would. She'd soon be off on her weekly visit to Westcott's Wildlife Park. Hence her bubbly mood: hence my flat one. She'd be out there striding around the zoo inspecting a range of interesting animals while I'd be in here shuffling round the ops table working my way through the speys, castrates and dentals – the only high point the abscess on a poodle's anal sphincter that was going to need lancing. Nothing to get my teeth into there – certainly not where the poodle's posterior was concerned.

Eric had warned me that Crystal tended to hog all the zoo work, and he was right. Since starting at Prospect House, I'd never got within a whisker of seeing the Wildlife Park. I was just left to wallow here and I was finding it a bit of a bore.

I managed a curt 'Morning' in reply before Crystal whizzed up to reception to confer with Beryl about her schedule for the day once she returned from the zoo. Then whoosh ... she was gone.

'Never mind, Paul,' said Beryl, giving me a sympathetic one-eyed look as I watched Crystal's car roar out of the drive. 'I've got Mr

Hargreaves coming in to see you this afternoon. You always find him a challenge.'

That was true. If I needed a client to light my fuse, then I guess Mr Hargreaves was the one most likely to put a match to it and put some sparkle in my life. I'd first met him a couple of months back when he was quick to inform me his hobby was herpetology and that he had a small collection of reptiles and amphibians. I expressed some interest – more as a PR exercise rather than as a genuine fascination for such creatures – but he took it to mean I was as enthusiastic as he was and began turning up time after time with some unusual species or other.

Unfortunately he had an irritating habit of always referring to them by their Latin names. Perhaps if I hadn't recognized his *Tarentola mauritanica* on that first encounter, he wouldn't have come back to see me, but I recognized it was a gecko and that impressed him. So, much to my consternation, the flow of reptiles and amphibians continued. Often he came in just for advice.

'I've got this *Pseudemys floridana* on approval. Do you think I should buy it?' His tall, twig-like body would bend over the table while I glumly watched some sort of terrapin splash about in a container of water.

'You'd better watch out for my *Hyla cinera*,' he said one day as he placed a clear plastic jar in front of me.

It appeared to contain nothing but a bunch of fresh leaves. Only when I unscrewed the lid and one of the leaves hopped onto the consulting table did I spot the tree frog. I didn't have to ask what was wrong as it flopped round in a circle, its right leg trailing behind it.

Mandy refused to handle it.

'No way,' she exclaimed, her chins wobbling, her rotund body all of a quiver. 'It gives me the creeps.' And she did just that by creeping out of the prep room.

'I'll do it myself then,' I said, and X-rayed the frog between hops. The radiograph revealed a fractured tibia which healed of its own accord without intervention from me.

Occasionally, Mr Hargreaves would bring in a more familiar animal.

'Here's my *Canis familiaris* for her booster,' he'd quip as Judy, his springer spaniel plodded in. But invariably there would be an accompanying exotic for my perusal. His *Trituris vulgaris* for example. It took me several minutes of searching the tangle of weeds in his aquarium before I spotted the newts.

That November afternoon he presented me with a real banger of a challenge. He slid the vivarium onto the consulting table. In it was a layer of sand, some small rocks and a log, its bark cracked, streaked silver and brown. I peered at the log intently, half-expecting it to slither away.

Mr Hargreaves chuckled. 'That's a real one. The *Trachysaurus rugosus* is underneath, probably buried in the sand.'

I placed a hand on the vivarium lid, stopped, wondered what sort of creature he was talking about, lost my nerve and said, 'You dig it out.'

Mr Hargreaves heaved his thin shoulders, spread out his stick-like arms. 'Just as you wish.' He lifted off the lid, pushed the log to one side and sank his bony fingers into the sand. A scaly, grey head poked out, slowly followed by the rest of the stump tailed skink's body. Mr Hargreaves levered it onto the table. 'Its innards seem to be coming out.'

Gingerly, I grasped the reptile round the neck, its rough, dry skin rasping on my fingers as I twisted it over. It wriggled and thrashed, its tail whipping from side to side. Any minute I expected the tail to be jettisoned across the room. Just under the tail base was a coil of red, glistening tissues. Bowels. The skink had a prolapsed rectum.

'Wondered if it was something like that,' said Mr Hargreaves.

I explained to him that to get the loops of bowel back in, the skink would have to have an anaesthetic and that it might not be too easy to do.

So it proved. The difficulty was not the actual anaesthetic but finding someone to assist in administering it.

'Honestly, Paul, I can't,' declared Mandy, adamant in her refusal to help. And her fear seemed genuine enough, her dark eyes full of apprehension and her chins quivering yet again. And Lucy? She too backed away muttering vague excuses about needing to exercise the dogs.

'They're just a load of namby-pambies,' said Eric, bouncing into the theatre, the ends of his white coat, as usual, swirling round his ankles. 'Give it here.' He rammed the skink's head into the face mask and spun the ether valve onto full.

The skink lay inert, not a tremor, not a flicker of its tail. Both Eric and I peered at it closely, our noses almost touching, as we tried to determine whether the reptile was breathing or not.

'Guess you'd better chance it, eh?' said Eric, when several minutes had ticked by and we were still waiting for some movement of the skink's chest. 'Go on. Shove the thermometer up the blighter's arse.'

I lubricated the loops of intestine with antibiotic cream and gently began to prise them back in, only using the thermometer when the last loop had slipped out of sight, pushing it into the rectum to ensure the intestines had completely inverted themselves.

'There, that wasn't so difficult, was it?' Eric declared smugly, and tossing the face mask onto the anaesthetic trolley, he reached over to turn off the ether valve. 'Well, I'll be damned.' His strawberry nose twitched, his face a glimmer under the dome of his skull. He turned to me with an apologetic look in his red-rimmed eyes. 'Seems I forgot to push the hood down on the ether bottle. Nothing was coming through except oxygen.'

He sprung round the operating table and placed a finger and thumb either side of the skink's body which still lay there, inert. 'It's cold. That's why it's so sluggish. Oh well, almost as good as an anaesthetic.' Avoiding my eyes, he flapped quickly out of the room.

Mr Hargreaves was extremely grateful. 'Please accept this little gift for your waiting room. It's a *Carausius morusus*.'

Not wishing to offend, I accepted the creature, handing it over to a reluctant Lucy to look after. It proved to be a prolific breeder and within weeks a notice had to be pinned to the board in the waiting-room saying 'Wanted. Good homes for baby stick insects.'

Beryl thought the incident with the skink hilarious and typical of Eric.

'Will have to find you some more exotics,' she declared, leaning against the open back door, cigarette in her mouth, hand cupped below it. Did the woman ever use an ashtray?

My thoughts turned to lions, camels, giraffes – the sort of thing Crystal would deal with over at Westcott's Wildlife Park. The sort of thing I'd like to deal with. In your dreams, Paul. Still, I knew Beryl was doing her best to keep my interests in exotics alive, and what she had me dealing with next was beyond the wildest of those dreams. In fact, it was an absolute nightmare.

'They have four lungs instead of two,' said its owner, Mr Thomson, glancing up, his eyes sharp like a terrier's.

'Really?' I replied, keeping a wide gap between me and the consulting table as the tarantula crawled across his hand.

'Yes. And their jaws work vertically instead of horizontally. Fascinating, don't you think?'

'Fascinating, yes....' I faltered, still keeping my distance.

The spider's black body nestled in Mr Thomson's huge calloused hand, the long, furry legs dangling over his fingers. I was thankful when he informed me he'd just bought the spider from the local pet shop and knowing I was interested in such creatures – his friend Mr Hargreaves had told him – thought I might like to take a look. He prodded it back into its plastic carrying box and lifted his Jack Russell onto the table.

'But it's Ben here who really needs seeing. His anal glands are giving him jip again.'

I squeezed them with great relief. But I wasn't so lucky on the next visit. This time there was no dog: only the wretched spider.

'I'm having problems with it,' confessed Mr Thomson, placing the white box on the table. 'Wondered if you could help.'

I gulped. 'I don't really know much about spiders. In fact, nothing at all. I don't think—'

Mr Thomson raised his hairy hand, the sleeve of his jacket straining over the swell of well-developed biceps. 'I'd like a professional opinion anyway.'

'Of course,' I demurred, as the biceps rippled.

He opened the box and the spider slithered onto the table. 'You don't have to be a vet to see it's not well.'

I had to agree. The tarantula lay on its back, its legs closed over its bulbous abdomen. If ever a spider looked sick, that tarantula did. But what the hell was I supposed to do with it. Listen to its chest? Palpate its abdomen? Take its temperature? Ah ... I marched over to the trolley and whipped the thermometer from its pot of disinfectant.

'Blimey,' gulped Mr Thomson, his eyes on stalks, 'you're not going to—'

'No ... no.' I shook my head. The intention was to use the thermometer to prod the spider, see if there were any signs of life. I was rewarded with a slight tremor of the legs. Unless the tarantula was doing a terminal knees-up, there was life in it yet. I flicked it over and gingerly examined it closer. The spider's coat of fine bristles had lost their black lustre. They looked lifeless, dry.

'Interesting,' I murmured, running the tip of the thermometer along its back. 'See? There seems to be a hairline crack down its back.' Something from my school biology days stirred in my memory. I turned to Mr Thomson. 'Has the spider been acting strange at all in the past couple of days?'

'In what way?'

'Well, for example, hiding under a stone or the like.'

'Now you come to mention it, yes it has. Thought it was 'cos it was ill.'

'It's no illness,' I said, straightening up. 'It's ecdysis.'

Mr Thomson's wind-etched features creased in concern. He scraped his hand across the dark stubble on his chin. 'Sounds serious.'

'No, not really. The tarantula's sloughing. As you may know, spiders don't have skeletons like us but moult, casting off their old exoskeletons.' My biology notes came flooding back. I spouted on, clearly impressing Mr Thomson. And myself.

He phoned the next day to confirm that the exoskeleton had completely split and a new, gleaming, altogether larger tarantula had crawled out.

'Just wait to you see him,' he said enthusiastically. 'He's huge.'

I shuddered, hoping that wait would be a very long time.

Meanwhile, Beryl wasn't waiting, bless her black woolly stockings. She seemed determined to whip up more exotics for me and I did wonder whether she was systematically going through the West Sussex telephone directories, cold-calling people to see if they had any unusual pets that needed treating.

It didn't surprise me when she rubbed her liver-spotted hands together, bounced up and down on her stool and crowed, 'Paul, I've got a treat in store for you. A Mr Patel is bringing in a snake.'

I felt my heart constrict as if a boa – and not of the feather variety – had already slid round it.

'I knew you'd be pleased,' she added.

Pleased? She thought I'd be pleased? What a load of cobras.

No one was around when Mr Patel turned up for his appointment. Funny that. Beryl was conveniently on the loo while Mandy and Lucy suddenly disappeared into the depths of Prospect House.

'You're all namby-pambies,' I said to myself, echoing Eric's sentiments. 'There's nothing to be scared of.' But then why were my legs trembling so much as I ushered Mr Patel in?

I'd had visions of a slim, brown-silk-skinned, turban-headed man, flute under one arm, carrying an Ali Baba basket, but that was just me being silly. The turbaned Mr Patel didn't have a flute. The Ali Baba basket he was carrying he lifted onto the consulting table and pushed towards me. In the absence of fluted music to entice out whatever was in the basket, I suggested Mr Patel did the honours with his hands.

'No sweat, mate,' he said in a breezy cockney accent and lifted the lid to pull out coil after coil of snake.

My throat went into spasm. 'Big isn't it,' I croaked and backed away as the snake weaved across the table towards me, knocking the basket to one side.

'Quite a size. Two point one metres to be precise. Though anacondas can grow much bigger.' Mr Patel grasped a coil of gleaming snake, its dark-green, black-spotted flanks twisting in his hands, dragging him onto the table. 'He's a strong lad,' he added, as he pulled at the snake making the table and snake lurch forward while I lurched back. 'Sid's a bit frisky. Should have put him in the fridge before coming: it would have quietened him down.' He jerked the snake's head away from my coat pocket.

Sid flicked out his tongue before, with a smooth, gliding movement, he slithered over Mr Patel's wrist and proceeded to advance up his arm, wrapping himself round and round as he inched up to his shoulder.

I didn't have to ask what was wrong: it was all too obvious. Protruding from Sid's mouth was a plug – an ordinary, white 13 amp three-pin plug.

'How come?' I asked, pointing a shaky finger.

'Not sure to be honest. But I think it was probably the rat I gave him last night. Guess some of the blood must have spilt on his heating pad.'

'You mean…?'

''Fraid so, mate. He's swallowed the pad. And I can't pull the damned thing out. See?' Mr Patel yanked at the plug, an inch of flex appeared; but no more. 'Bugger, ain't it?'

'Stop,' I said hastily. 'You might rip his stomach open.'

'Me thinks you might have to do that to get it out.'

'Maybe,' I murmured, desperately trying to decide what to do for the best. Anacondas and the like were well known for being able to devour whole pigs in one go. The heating pad would be a mere snack in comparison. 'How long was the flex.'

Mr Patel scratched his turban. 'Oh … must have been about a metre or so.'

'And you say Sid's about two metres plus. Uhmmm. Well there's an outside chance the pad could pass through.'

'But with the plug on, surely not?'

'No. No. I'll snip that off,' I said and reached for the nail scissors.

Beryl flew off her perch when Mr Patel re-entered reception with his creaking basket and it was left to me to book an appointment for a week's time.

The situation hadn't changed much when next I saw him except that the flex had now disappeared.

'Well, at least it must be moving through,' I commented. But I wasn't too happy. Sid was due for another of his weekly meals but so far had turned his nose up at the rat that had been offered him. 'Let's get an X-ray just to see what's going on.'

'More like what's going through, eh?' joked Mr Patel, sounding remarkably unperturbed by the whole incident, as I ushered him into the waiting-room.

'Who's going to help?' My question echoed down an empty corridor. Somewhere I heard the clatter of feet and a door slam. There was a muffled cough behind the closed door of the office. Oh, so we were all playing hide-and-seek now, were we? Peek-a-boo. I've a snake for you.

There was the skid of tyres on the gravel, the roar of an engine dying. Sounded like Crystal had arrived back from visiting one of her special clients.

'So what have you got there Paul?' she asked, sailing into reception and looking at the wicker basket I was about to drag down to the X-ray room. 'Your washing?'

The basket hissed and rattled. I explained.

'He sounds a bit lively to me,' said Crystal. 'Perhaps we ought to pop him in the fridge for a while. Get him cooled down a bit and then get him X-rayed. I'd be happy to help. Haven't seen an anaconda in ages.'

Well, this was a first, having Crystal help me out. Go for it, Paul. Go for it. I did, clearing space in the fridge and squeezing the basket between the shelves before returning to the office to find Crystal talking to Beryl. She broke off her conversation as I entered. 'Beryl tells me you've been seeing quite a few exotics lately,' she said, smiling at me. Ah, that smile. Those rosy lips. That cupid bow. So like a … prolapsed rectum sprang to mind. Oh really, Paul. That's disgusting.

'You've had a skink with a prolapsed rectum,' Crystal was saying.

'Oh, yes,' I said, taking a deep breath. Get a grip, man.

'And a tarantula.'

I nodded, looking across at Beryl who had turned a whiter shade of pale. Spiders, snakes and the like were definitely not her cup of tea. Talking of which....

'Good idea,' said Crystal when Beryl suggested making one. 'I'd love a cup.'

The scream that emanated from the kitchen had both Crystal and I leaping from our seats. Oh my God. Beryl. Our thoughts were as one. Tea ... milk ... fridge ... snake.... Beryl staggered in, trembling like jelly, a hand covering the right side of her face.

'Here, sit down,' said Crystal, easing her down into a chair.

'It was such a shock,' uttered Beryl, shaking her head. 'I opened the fridge door and there it was. Coiled round the semi-skimmed. I just didn't expect it.'

'No, of course not,' said Crystal. 'You can blame me for that. It was my idea. So sorry.' She put an arm round Beryl's shoulder and patted it. 'Can I get you anything?'

Beryl, the hand still covering half her face said, 'I wouldn't mind a cigarette.' She looked up at Crystal with her good eye. 'If that's all right with you.'

I saw Crystal's arm quickly retract from her shoulder. Wow. Beryl was pushing her luck a bit. There was a strictly 'No Smoking' policy in the hospital – and Beryl knew it. Guess she was just playing the sympathy card. It worked.

'I'll get your bag,' said Crystal, after a moment's hesitation. 'Up in reception is it?'

'Ah that's better,' sighed Beryl once she'd lit up. She tilted her head back and a plume of smoke poured from each nostril. She might have felt better but she certainly didn't look better. There was still fear etched in her face. A sort of wildness. For a moment I couldn't put my finger on it. There was no trembling. That had stopped. Her complexion had returned to its normal pan-pasted colour. No, it was something about the eyes. Yes, that was it. The eyes. Or, to be more precise, the whites of the eyes. Or, to be even more precise, the white of her right eye. That was all one could see: a ball of white.

I remember Eric telling me over a drink at the Woolpack that when unduly stressed, Beryl's false eye was liable to drop out. Had the sight of the snake precipitated such a fall-out? Was her glass eye at that moment rolling around the kitchen? Or worse still, had it fallen in the milk and was now rattling around the bottom of the carton?

Crystal had also noticed and was staring slack-jawed.

I leaned forward and studied Beryl's face more intently, deciding that the eyeball was still *in situ* after all. Only it had swivelled back to front.

'What are you gawping at?' she snapped, jerking her head back. It was an action that caused the glass eye to rotate back into partial view. It gave Beryl a severe sharp-angled squint as if she was attempting to peer up her right nostril.

'Er ... nothing ... nothing ...' I muttered. 'Just seeing if you were OK.' I hadn't the courage to look her in the eye – her good one – and tell her. She'd have to see for herself later.

'OK then,' said Crystal, looking at her watch, 'let's get cracking on that snake before appointments start.'

The anaconda was half out of the basket, draped across a couple of packs of dog meat, but the coolness of the fridge had quickly brought it to a halt. Between us we hiked out the coils of snake and arranged them in a heap on the X-ray table.

'This is going to be a bit of guesswork,' said Crystal, stretching Sid out and pushing an X-ray plate under him, sliding it up and down. 'Any ideas, Paul?'

Hey. What was this? Crystal asking me? Snakes alive. This was another first. I put a hand on either side of the snake's flanks, starting at the neck end, gradually working my way down, gently squeezing as I went. Two-thirds of the way down I felt what I thought was some resistance. Could have been the heating pad. Whatever, it was a starting point for X-raying. It took three plates before the pad was eventually highlighted.

Crystal stood in front of the X-ray clipped to the viewing screen, finger and thumb under her chin. 'So what do you think? Do you want to operate?'

Hey. She was at it again. Crystal Sharpe, veterinary surgeon *par excellence*, asking me for my views. Me. An assistant who had barely progressed from expressing anal glands, now being asked to express his opinions. I was tempted to say 'Yes. Let's operate.' After all it would have been fascinating to carry out surgery on a snake – especially one of this size. But I hesitated. Could that just be self-interest. What about the interests of Sid? It would be much better for him if we could avoid operating. 'Liquid paraffin often works wonders,' I found myself saying.

Crystal swung round and looked at me. Oh those cornflower-blue eyes again. That delicate scent which filled my nostrils. I recoiled - much as the anaconda was starting to do as he warmed up.

'You reckon it's worth a try then,' she said. 'Uhmm.... OK. Fair enough. Now where are those nurses. Never around when you want them.' She strode out in to the corridor and called, 'Mandy?'

There was a faint reply from the direction of the dispensary. 'Coming.'

When Mandy appeared, Crystal ordered her to help carry the anaconda into the operating theatre. I was flabbergasted when she uttered a meek 'Certainly' and picked up a length of Sid without batting one of those long, dark eyelashes of hers. And to think she'd been so squeamish about the tree frog and Skink. Moreover she didn't flinch when Crystal asked her to prise open the snake's jaw while I was shown how to insert a stomach tube down Sid's oesoph agus and syringe in ten millilitres of liquid paraffin. Not a murmur not a squeak out of her. I could happily have squeezed a coil of Sid around her neck.

A three-day wait followed. I felt the strain and I'm sure Sid did as well – especially when he passed the heating pad. Within twenty-four hours, his appetite had returned and a rat had been devoured. Mr Patel was over the moon.

'And guess what, mate,' he exclaimed. 'I tried putting another plug on the heating pad ... just on the off-chance.'

'And...?'

'It still works.'

Crystal was also pleased at the outcome. 'You made the right deci sion not to operate. It would have been risky.'

I squirmed in Sid-like fashion. But when she went on to say there were a couple of interesting cases that had cropped up at the Wildlife Park and would I like to take a look at them with her some time, I almost tied myself in knots.

Beryl cawed with alarm and nearly toppled from her perch when I wrapped my arms around her, gave her a squeeze and told her the news. Sure, I had a crush on Crystal, but it was Beryl I had to thank

Chapter 15

I'm not sure when I was first asked the question but I've a feeling it was soon after I'd started at Prospect House, back in June. Heavens, was that really only six months? Seems aeons ago. And the person who asked it was Mrs Paget. Ah, yes, dear Cynthia Paget – the lady with whom I had lodged. The lady who saw me struggling to cope with the rigours of practice and offered to help by allowing me extra time in her kitchen – not to mention extra freezer space. She'd asked me to have a look at Chico – that little chihuahua of hers – now dead, a casualty of a road accident. Back then the only casualty was my heels. If I'd been an angel, the place where I'd have feared to tread most would have been in Mrs Paget's hallway as I was constantly being nipped there by Chico.

Mrs Paget, in her loose-fitting, pink, quilted housecoat, suggested I examined Chico in her bedroom. 'He's much calmer on my bed. It'll be easier to see what's up,' she explained, her housecoat slipping down a few inches. I wasn't having any of it – well certainly not from the likes of Mrs Paget. He and not she found himself being manhandled in the sitting-room where overgrown nails were clipped and the only thing bared were the usual teeth.

'Had I always wanted to do it?' she asked, as the last nail clawed its way across the carpet.

The question was also asked by Mandy. It was when I was deep inside a Great Dane bitch trying to locate her reproductive organs.

Same with Lucy in bed one evening (different place, similar position).

And the answer? Yes. I'd always wanted to be a vet – well, at least since I was ten years old.

At that time we lived in Nigeria, my father an army officer. In our large, corrugated red-roofed bungalow with its sprawling compound,

I amassed a large menagerie of pets. No surprise that my favourite book was Gerald Durrell's *My Family and Other Animals*. I too had my animals: a cat called Sooty, three tortoises, some rats, five ducks, several chickens, an African Grey parrot called Polly, a monkey – the species of which I never did find out – and, most treasured of all, Poucher – a Labrador-cross with the sweetest temperament you could ever have wished for.

I'll never forget the time she went missing. For three days we lived in fear that she'd been attacked by some wild animal and was lying out in the bush slowly dying. We searched high and low but found no sign of her. She eventually crawled home, her right leg nearly torn off at the thigh. The army doctor saved her, patiently stitching up the muscles, tendons and skin while I stood by and watched. Riveted to the spot. Fascinated. And as I nursed her back to health, encouraged her to take her first meal, helped her to limp round the garden, saw in the dark-brown eyes, the trust she put in me, I knew I couldn't possibly do anything else with my life other than take the path that beckoned: the path that led to becoming a vet.

Of course I didn't put it quite like that to Mrs Paget otherwise I'd have had her falling at my feet, kissing them as Chico bit them.

But I had achieved my ambition.

So was this it? Rummaging around Cynthia Paget, clipping the nails of her vicious chihuahua? Yes, well. Maybe I still had to reach my peak. And to judge from Mrs Paget's heaving bosom, she clearly hoped I'd have a peek at hers.

One client who'd had ambitions to scale the same heights but had backed down at an early stage was Miss Millichip.

'Always wanted to be a vet,' she declared. 'Ever since I was a mere slip of a girl.'

I couldn't picture Mildred Millichip as a mere slip of anything. But the laws of nature being what they are meant that once she must have been young. Someone must have conceived her. Someone must have allowed her in the world. Someone must have gathered her up in their arms and loved her. I'm sure someone did. But it was hard to imagine who that someone might have been.

Could she ever have had shiny plaits or a glossy pony-tail I wonder, gazing now at her wiry, grey straggle of hair like a discarded scouring pad, tied back with an elastic band and a couple of broken-toothed combs? And were those grey eyes ever innocent and trusting as they now stared back at me like two torpedoes ready to fire, echoed by the raft of grey on a protruding upper lip? No one could say she was pretty. Her looks caught your eye rather like a thorn snags your sock.

'Only the war intervened,' she continued.

First or second? I thought.

'Put a stop to everything. Career, the lot.' She sliced a set of square-nailed fingers through the air. 'All got the chop. But we had to do our duty. I was in the tank corps you know.'

No surprise there. She was built like one.

'And after the war … well … I landed up here.'

'At least you've got your animals,' I ventured to say.

Indeed Miss Millichip had a whole battalion of them – putting my Nigerian menagerie to shame. She lived in a post-war bungalow she shared with a multitude of cats and odd stray dogs; but most of her time was spent in one or other of the many outbuildings which housed the main bulk of her brood.

It was through Beryl – who else? – that I first met her earlier that summer. The receiver was waved at me when I arrived for work one Wednesday morning. Could I visit a Miss Millichip?

'Ask her to come in.'

Beryl's eye widened in horror and, hand clasped over the receiver, said in a loud whisper, 'Not Mildred Millichip. She never comes in.'

I'd been told that practice policy was to encourage appointments rather than visits. So if that was the case … I snatched the phone from Beryl.

'Mr Mitchell here. I gather you want a visit.'

'Mr Mitchell. I don't think I know you.'

'I'm new here.'

'Oh in that case put me on to Dr Sharpe.'

'I'm afraid she's not here.'

'When will she be back?'

'When she's finished her match' would have been the truthful reply as it was Crystal's tennis morning. 'This afternoon. But she's booked up with appointments,' I said.

There was a loud tut. 'And Mr Sharpe? I doubt if he's booked up. He'll have to do I suppose.' The tone was distinctly unenthusiastic.

Eric was at the dentist's. I saw Beryl hold up her hands, rocking them from side to side in unison with shaking her head whilst at the same time silently mouthing 'No! No! No!' She looked like she was auditioning for *Guys and Dolls*. Clearly I was in danger of rocking the boat if Eric and Miss Millichip were on board together. 'He's unavailable,' I said. Beryl sat down with relief.

'You'll have to do then,' said Miss Millichip, her voice sounding distinctly disappointed.

'What's the problem?'

'The greyhounds' got canker.'

'Can't you bring him in?'

There was a sharp intake of breath. 'What do you think I am? Some sort of American bus service? It's my greyhounds. All eight of them.'

That set the tone for a track record of visits. Whenever she phoned demanding one, I'd be trapped into making it. You could bet on it every time.

On that visit, as on subsequent ones, I had problems finding her in the maze of sheds, lean-tos and outhouses that encircled her bungalow. I never discovered her in the house actually sitting, putting her feet up. Her feet were always firmly entrenched in green gumboots, plastered in mud, striding from building to building.

She could be in the kennels housing her greyhounds and beagles or in the stables with her three Welsh ponies. Failing that, there were the hen houses and duck quarters; and if not in there, then in the pigsties tending to Gert and Daisy, her Yorkshire saddleback pigs.

Central to this conglomeration of buildings, adjoining the tackroom, was a small shed which she called her 'brain centre'. An office of sorts, it was littered with paper. Charts of pig growth curves hung, faded and lopsided from the walls. A curling, year-at-a-glance calendar given to her by a veterinary drug company, its logo emblazoned across the top, was festooned with multi-coloured pins and scribbled names. Bessie, Babs, Clarence and many more, signalled the dates that bitches were mated, dates they were due, intermingled with farrowing sows, calving cows and dates booked for the blacksmith and A.I. man. It looked like some coded battle plan from World War Two with Miss Millichip the commander-in-chief, the only person capable of unscrambling it all.

Along the opposite wall ranged a series of shelves, bowed down under the weight of a motley collection of ancient books and journals. *Hodders Guide to Animal Husbandry* was one title I picked out – 1961, second edition. Another was *General Principles of Animal Nursing*. Its sepia pages could have proudly graced the shelves of the

Science Museum's library. But one book above all – a book that Mildred Millichip constantly referred to – was an old veterinary dictionary, long since superseded by later editions. The binding was cracked, pages cellotaped in, others dog-eared from constant use. And that was the problem – the constant use. Miss Millichip was always quoting this dictionary, always looking up medical conditions, always trying the suggested remedies.

'My bible,' she'd say, forgetting her bible was an edition more appropriate for treating the ailments of the animals as they emerged from the ark rather than administering to the needs of modern live-stock.

The greyhounds with the ear problems were a good example.

'Canker,' declared Miss Millichip in a no-nonsense, don't chal-lenge-me tone of voice. She'd hoisted one of the greyhounds onto a table in what she called her 'inspection shed' where the poor creature sat trembling, head tilted to one side. When the dog's hind leg came up in an attempt to dig at her ear, Miss Millichip's hand shot out to ram the leg down.

'Stop that, Gemima,' she boomed. Both dog and I flinched.

Besides my usual black bag, I'd brought a small leather case containing a set of instruments for looking at eyes and ears. I was particularly proud of this set – precision made in Germany, expensive and brand new. Time spent peering unclearly into the murky depths of dogs' ears was now a thing of the past. With the aid of my gleaming auriscope, I could scan those canals, now sufficiently well illuminated and magnified, to make diagnosis of any ear problem an easy task.

Well in theory anyway.

Aware that Miss Millichip's torpedo eyes were trained on me, I made a show of snapping open the case, picking out the auriscope base and clipping on the head containing bulb and magnifying lens. I now had to attach a cone from a choice of four, varying in size according to the size of the ear canal being examined.

'Now let's see,' I said aloud, 'which one would be most suitable for Gemima.' My fingers hovered over the cones. I felt like a little schoolboy deciding on which sweetie to choose. Will I ever grow up?

There was a loud sniff from Miss Millichip.

'This one, I think,' I continued, lifting out the largest with an exaggerated flourish. Boy, was I showing off.

There was another disapproving sniff from Miss Millichip. 'Haven't got time for all that fancy gadgetry,' she said.

'Ah, but having the proper equipment does help one reach the correct diagnosis,' I replied (pompous prat) and waved the auriscope at her like a magician about to perform some wonderful trick.

'No need. I've already told you what it is. Canker.'

'We'll soon find out.' I advanced on the trembling greyhound and lifted her right ear. She winced and pulled away. 'So this is the bad one is it?'

'They both hurt,' said Miss Millichip, edging round the table to clamp the dog's head firmly to her bosom. 'Now hold still, Gemima, while the vet pokes his newfangled contraption down your ear.'

'It's called an auriscope,' I informed her.

'Well, whatever. Just see how bad the canker is.'

I switched the instrument so that the bulb illuminated the cone, gently lifted the flap of Gemima's ear and eased the tip of the cone in. I peered down. Nothing. I eased the cone up a little and slid it back in. Still nothing. A blank wall. Literally that. A solid wall of white.

'Your gadget playing up then?' queried Miss Millichip.

'I'm not sure....' I eased the auriscope out. The tip of the cone was caked in a clump of wet, chalky material. No wonder I couldn't see down it. 'What's this?' I waved the cone at Miss Millichip.

'Your horiscope or whatever you call it.'

'No. The muck on the end of it.'

'Bit of my canker treatment by the looks of it,' she said, peering at the end of the cone as I pushed it under her nose. 'Boracic acid powder, twice daily. As recommended in my dictionary for the treatment of mites.'

I winced, resisting the urge to shove the cone up her nose. Now, now, Paul, that's not professional. Keep cool. 'But it hasn't worked, has it?'

'My dictionary says it should.'

I fought to keep my voice from rising. 'But it hasn't, has it?'

'Well, the dogs do seem a bit quieter since I started the treatment. So maybe it's had some effect.'

Quieter eh? I thought. Probably because they couldn't hear themselves bark with all that stuff rammed in their ears. But it wouldn't have killed off the ear mites if they were present unless the sheer volume of powder Miss Millichip had been pouring in had suffocated them. 'Look, first we need to syringe Gemima's ears out. The same applies to your other dogs.'

'I'll get some soapy water with a pinch of washing soda in it.'

'Er, I don't think that's wise. Soapy water on red raw ear canals …'
I shook my head. 'Gemima would hit the roof.'

'But my dictionary says—'

I interrupted, 'Forget your dictionary. There's a new preparation
I use to clean out the ear canals so that the mites can then be treated.'

Miss Millichip glanced up at the dictionary on her bookshelf.

'No, you won't find it in there,' I added firmly. 'But it does work.
Honest. Let me show you.'

Ten minutes later, I'd excavated all the compressed powder that
had been shovelled down Gemima's ear canals. Another check with
the auriscope revealed a thriving colonies of mites. 'Now use this,' I
said, handing over a small plastic bottle of anti-parasitic solution. 'A
good squirt down each ear and massage well in.'

Miss Millichip peered dubiously at the bottle – it looked lost in
her massive hand. 'This won't go far. Most of my dogs and half the
cats are scratching or shaking their heads. My dictionary says I
should treat the lot.'

For once I agreed with her dictionary. A litre of mange dressing
was ordered from the local wholesalers. Miss Millichip looked it up
in her dictionary. Yes. The dressing was mentioned. So she was
happy to use it.

A week later she was on the phone again. Beryl waved me over.
'It's Mildred Millichip,' she whispered loudly. 'She wants another
visit.'

'Well, Crystal's around. She can go. After all that's who she wanted
in the first place.'

'Not any more. She wants you. Seems she was impressed by your
horiscope.' Beryl pulled a what-on-earth-does-she-mean? face. But
she booked the visit when I nodded. As I explained to her later – no,
Miss Millichip hadn't read my palm, got out the Tarot cards or gazed
into a crystal ball. But I wish she had. Then I might have been
prepared for what was to come.

I'd rung the bell on the front door of the bungalow several times.
I could hear it buzzing away deep inside. But no one came. I guessed
Miss Millichip was probably round the back somewhere – that somewhere being the maze of outbuildings that stretched through the acre
or so of garden. Several greyhounds came bounding out into their
runs from the long, wooden poultry shed which housed their kennels.
They leapt up at the mesh fencing, tails wagging, barking furiously.

I'd been about to call out for Miss Millichip, but it seemed pointless to try and compete against the cacophony of barks and howls that had now erupted. I expected the racket to have drawn Miss Millichip from whichever building she happened to be in. But there was still no sign of her. Really this was not good news. My time was precious: I shouldn't be hunting the woman down. She should be here to meet me. Beginning to feel cross, I marched over to the so-called office, the door of which was open. That old veterinary dictionary – the red tattered one – lay open on the table. No doubt Miss Millichip had been genning up before doing battle with me.

I stepped out and round to the stables where the three Welsh cobs looked up from their hay nets and gave a wicker of greeting. Still no sign of her. Chickens flapped and squawked, jumping away from me as I slithered down the muddy path towards the pig-sty. The noise of the hounds had abated somewhat so I stopped, cleared my throat and shouted, 'Miss Millichip.' A crow cawed in the field beyond. A couple of ducks came running up, quacking, looking for scraps. Still no answer. I tried again. 'Miss Millichip.'

Two heads appeared round the corner of the pig-sty; porky eyes peered at me; several grunts were uttered; then, with a squeal from each of them, the two saddlebacks trotted to the centre of their mud-bath of a paddock and turned to stare at me, jowls chomping, froth and flecks of red bubbling round their snouts.

My heart skipped a beat. Just what was that around their lips? That red foam? Blood? I picked my way over to the sty's fence for a closer look. The pigs gave another loud snort and swung away. It was then I heard the moan. A long soft moan coming from inside the sty. I could feel my heart thumping against my chest as I clung to the fence to prevent myself slipping in the sea of mud which had oozed through from the paddock and made the path up to the sty treacherous. There was another moan as I reached the wall of the sty and peered over, dreading what I might find. And my worst fears were realized.

There lay Miss Millichip, sprawled on the muddy concrete, half-conscious, neck twisted to one side, a gash on her temple, and half her face eaten away.

Of course, it made banner headlines in the *Westcott Gazette*. YOUNG VET SAVES LADY'S BACON – full report on page three. There it was given a good half-page with a photo of me grinning nervously next to Gert and Daisy and another of me looking equally nervous next to a head-bandaged Miss Millichip in hospital.

As it turned out, my initial impression of Miss Millichip's features being torn from her face by two rampaging pigs had been a little wide of the mark. A little too Grand Guignol. True, she had gashed her head open when she'd slipped in their pen. And true, Gertie and Daisy had investigated, snuffling at her bloody wound. When asked my veterinary opinion as to whether they would have made a meal of her, well, there seemed no harm in suggesting that it could have happened.

'So,' said the young reporter, 'if you hadn't turned up when you did it would have been chips for her.'

Indeed. Millichips I thought to myself. But said nothing aloud for fear of being quoted. Wouldn't do to ham things up too much.

Of course the publicity generated was good for the practice. There seemed to be a sudden surge in new clients with much whispering of 'That's him ... there', and nudging of elbows as I walked through the waiting-room riding high on my new-found fame – nothing like hogging the limelight – until I overheard someone saying 'He's the pig man. Hmm ... looks like one too.' That soon brought me back to earth with a bump.

As for Miss Millichip, what could I say? Well actually I could have said virtually anything. She was so, so grateful for what I had done. Not that she necessarily took any notice of what I said. That depended whether it tallied with her bible – that red, battered out-of-date veterinary dictionary of hers.

When she'd recovered and was back at her bungalow, the battle between the gospel according to Paul – Paul Mitchell that is – and the faith that she gained from her dictionary recommenced. An unholy war of words would erupt on every subsequent visit.

'Jasper's coat feels very greasy,' I said, having just given a greyhound his booster vaccination while holding up his scruff. I looked at my fingers, sliding them together.

'I've been rubbing olive oil into his skin,' stated Miss Millichip. 'My dictionary says it's the best way to treat dandruff.'

I glanced at my watch. There was still time to explain the problems of seborrhoea before I had to get back for evening surgery. I left Miss Millichip leafing through her dictionary to S for Skin, a bottle of medicated shampoo on the table beside her.

On another occasion one of her beagles suffered for a fortnight with a sore eye. Miss Millichip had been bathing it with strained weak tea.

'Doesn't seem to be getting any better,' she admitted, when she eventually called me in.

The poor beagle had very puffy eyelids with severe reddening of the lining, the corners stained brown with tears. The centre of the eye was white and pitted.

'What's that green stuff?' asked Miss Millichip, watching me suspiciously as I instilled some drops into the dog's eye.

'Fluorescein. It will show us if there's any ulceration there.'

'Jasper's just got a cold in his eye. That's what it says in my dictionary.'

'Oh really?' I replied, turning the Beagle's head towards her. The fluorescein had clearly delineated the crater pitting the surface of the cornea. 'Does your dictionary tell you what that is – U for ulcer?' She was given a tube of antibiotic ointment to put in the eye three times a day. 'And no more tea,' I snapped, as she glanced up at the bookshelf.

The final showdown came that December when Miss Millichip's greyhounds and beagles erupted in a frenzy of scratching and biting at themselves. The result was dogs with angry red spots on their abdomens and legs; and large areas of raw skin, seeping, the hair in those areas rubbed away.

The annunciation made by Miss Millichip via her bible (veterinary dictionary) was E for Eczema. 'Classic symptoms,' she boomed.

Not that damned book again I thought as I completed the examination of twelve very itchy dogs.

In each case, I only had to run my finger lightly along one of their flanks for a back leg to shoot up and start clawing at the skin. A very strong scratch reflex. But what was causing the irritation? F for fleas? But there were no signs of flea dirts. M for mange? The lesions weren't typical. My mental dictionary was beginning to let me down. I needed to come up with a diagnosis ASAP before I became S for stumped.

As we walked back across the yard from the kennels, I stopped to peer into a shed full of straw bales.

'I suppose you've tried treating the dogs?' I asked, leaning over the door to pick up a handful of straw. Silly question. The answer was bound to be 'Yes'.

'Of course. Chopped parsley, garlic pills and boiled fish. Internal cleansing. Does the world of good.' Miss Millichip saw my look. S for sceptical. 'Well, it can often help,' she added.

'But not in this case,' I said, throwing down the straw and smacking my hands together to shake off the dust.

'I'm now trying Simpson's Blood Mixture. My dictionary recommends it to cool the blood.'

'An F word would be the best thing for this lot.'

'You what? An F word?' exclaimed Miss Millichip, visibly startled. I swear that wasn't in her bible.

'F for fire. Put a match to all this straw.'

'But I couldn't possibly do that,' she protested. 'It's the straw for the dogs' bedding. I've only just bought it. Cost me a packet.'

'Cost you more than a packet if you persist in using it. Your dogs will end up with chronic skin damage.'

'But why?'

'The straw's alive with forage mites. They're causing all the itchiness. Burn the lot of it.'

Miss Millichip opened her mouth to protest again.

'Mildred, burn it,' I repeated. 'It will save you a great deal in vet's bills.'

That struck a cord. A match was struck too and the straw got burnt.

'I also burnt that old veterinary dictionary,' she later told me.

I couldn't believe my ears. 'You did what, Mildred?'

'You heard. Burnt it.'

Wow! So Miss Millichip had finally got rid of that wretched dictionary. I felt like a punch-drunk priest on hearing the news. 'You can't imagine how pleased I am to hear you say that,' I confessed.

Thank God. Now there'd be no more ancient remedies inflicted on the animals, and Miss Millichip would at last accept my advice without constantly referring to that battered old book of hers. But hang on. What's this she's saying?

'I must admit it was rather out-of-date. So I decided it was time I bought the latest edition.' She waved a glossy pristine book at me. 'My new bible.'

At the sight of it, my feelings rapidly became very unchristian.

So I got out of there PDQ – pretty damned quick.

Chapter 16

'What planet are you on?'

I didn't reply.

'Paul ... hello ... anyone at home?' Lucy leaned across the sofa and prodded me.

'Sorry. Miles away.'

'Exactly. Several thousand light years away by the look of you.' Lucy sat back and redirected her gaze at the TV screen where a lioness was stalking through the parched grass of a Kenyan Game Park approaching the edge of a lake for a drink. 'I thought you liked these wildlife programmes.'

True I did. And true I had been watching this one. But as that lioness had drifted through the wildlife park my mind had drifted to our own wildlife park here in Wescott. Yes I know. There was no real comparison. The grass here was more bowling green than savannah; Westcott's lake more for toy boats than slaking the thirst of a lion; and any crocodiles seen would be the lines of schoolchildren passing through.

I blamed it all on Crystal. I'd lost count of the number of times I had scaled mountains in the Austrian Tyrol since I'd first set eyes on those gorgeous blue eyes and Julie Andrews features. But ever since she'd mentioned us visiting Westcott's Wildlife Park together I'd been up the Limpopo without a paddle. But even if I'd had a paddle I'd still have been oar-struck at the thought of striding through the reserve with Crystal at my side in a crisp khaki safari jacket, tight jodphurs, and knee-length boots, tracking down an injured rhino here, a battered buffalo there, ever wary of the danger that could be lurking behind the next acacia tree – or rather weeping willow – as we're still talking Westcott here – where even if the trail's hot (and getting more hot and sticky by the minute as my imagination takes fire) the climate's certainly not.

So we continue to thrash through the bush (rhododendrons) – to emerge at the lakeside (edge of pond) to take in the broad sweep of water (pond again) – the raucous cry of the fish eagle (seagull) and the sight of a pack of hyenas (two dachshunds and a Yorkshire terrier) loping across the parched yellowed grass (there'd been a hosepipe ban all summer) so typical of this part of Kenya (West Sussex).

I felt another prod.

'Paul. Why have you got that silly expression on your face? What's wrong with you?'

Of course when the visit to Westcott's Wildlife Park finally materialized it was nothing like I'd imagined. Crystal in tight white jodhpurs? In your dreams, Paul. Nevertheless she was dressed for the occasion; well-cut dark-green corduroy jeans, a chunky polo-neck sweater and puffa-style light-green gilet. It was certainly enough to get my bongos beating.

Not so Westcott's Wildlife Park. I'm not sure what I expected. An expanse of undulating paddocks through which roamed herds of antelope, zebra, a sprinkling of giraffes, set against a backcloth of the green slopes of the Downs? The reality was a fenced off corner of the municipal gardens across from the seafront, crammed with an ill-assorted collection of pens, paddocks and aviaries containing an even more ill-assorted collection of animals, of which the only one present in sufficient numbers to constitute a herd was the guinea pig.

I guess one could have passed a pleasant summer's afternoon strolling through the municipal gardens, admiring the beds of purple petunias, the rows of orange marigolds, the reds of adjacent salvias – the kaleidoscope of clashing colours enough to send you reeling off to the pavilion for a cup of stewed tea drunk from a white plastic cup. If the sight of white-flannelled or pleated-skirted legs bent at the knees and buttocks in bowls-mode didn't do for you then you could roll up at Westcott's Wildlife Park and for £1.20 a time – £1.00 for pensioners – wander through its herds of rodents.

The day Crystal and I chose to visit, gauzy veils of sea mist had drifted in to saturate the gardens, coat the lawns in silver and hang in heavy folds through the branches of bare trees. The double gates to the Wildlife Park were bolted and chained, the place clearly closed.

Now out-of-season, it seemed that, from the information provided on a nearby noticeboard, if you wanted to walk on the wild side you could only do it on Wednesday afternoons, Saturdays and Sundays October–March.

Crystal drove past the gates and turned down a tarmac track marked 'Private' through a tunnel of rhododendrons that gave way to a substantial yard, dominated on one side by a huge mobile home – all gleaming chrome and aluminium. With the forest of aerials and satellite dishes that adorned its roof, it looked as if it had just dropped in from outer space. The adjacent prefabricated building looked very drab and mundane – single storey, painted green – an office block to judge from the bell and adjacent notice which read 'Ring' and 'Please Enter'.

Not that we had to ring. As we got out of the car, we were greeted by a series of howls that echoed through the trees. Wolves? A touch of Transylvania? Was a pack about to suddenly burst through the fog-bound trees? No. Though the two Alsatians that came bounding round from the side of the mobile home, teeth bared, drooling saliva, were just as scary.

'Hey now, you two, pack it in,' said Crystal, holding out her arm to allow the dogs to sniff her hand. They immediately quietened down with a whimper and pushed themselves against her thighs. Oh to be an Alsatian at that moment.

The man who appeared soon after the dogs was equally savage-looking but more in a Wild-Man-of-Borneo sort of way. Wild of hair – a mass of grey and black curls that looked desperate to tear themselves away from his scalp; matched by a shaggy unkempt beard and crumpled clothes that looked as if they'd been slept in for years. Rumpelstiltskin had nothing on this man. Peering out of the tangle of hair were two pebble-black eyes distorted through glasses, worn at the end of his nose, with lenses so murky I was tempted to trace 'clean me' across them.

Crystal introduced him. 'Paul, this is Kevin Winters, head keeper here.'

We shook hands.

'Paul is our new assistant,' she went on.

'Being shown the ropes, eh?' said Kevin with a smile which caused his lips to pucker out and expose a gap between his upper teeth through which his reply whistled. 'Well, there's plenty here to give you a challenge. There's Cleo for starters.'

As Crystal and I donned overalls and wellies I learnt that Cleo was a camel – a dromedary – the one with one hump.

'She's a bit of a bugger at the best of times,' said Kevin. 'But now he's gone lame she's certainly got the hump.' He shook his head and exhaled sharply, his breath whistling through the gap in his teeth like a kettle on the boil, the effect enhanced by the cloud of vapour which steamed into the damp air above him.

'As you say, Kevin. Nothing like a challenge,' said Crystal. She handed me a pack of surgical instruments from the back of the car, lifted out her black bag and closed the boot with a loud thud. 'OK, let's get cracking.'

Oh yes, please, Crystal. Where's your whip?

We followed Kevin in single file down a narrow muddy track through the rhododendrons and emerged onto a gravel path that ran alongside a row of aviaries containing budgerigars, some screeching cockatiels and a moth-eaten mynah. As we passed the bird I half-expected it to call out 'What's your name?' Cedric-style. Instead it looked up and said 'See yer later' followed by a Kevin-like whistle.

The path continued round an open enclosure where two Thomson gazelles, with their distinctive black flank stripes were grazing, their tails constantly flick, flick, flicking while an ostrich paced up and down the perimeter fence behind them.

The camel's pen was next door with an open-sided barn in which Cleo was bedded down in a deep pile of straw. She was chewing the cud, her lower lip swinging from side to side, her gaze directed away from us, across the muddy pen as if in a trance – perhaps dreaming of lost Arabian nights. She slowly swung her head in our direction as we approached the barn gate and gave us a haughty look, flicking her long eyelashes at us. I noticed she had a head collar on. So at least she could be handled – or so I thought.

Once inside the pen, we picked our way over to her, stopping when Kevin put out a restraining hand saying, 'I shouldn't get any closer if I were you. She's liable to spit.' Certainly enough froth had built up round Cleo's lips to do a cappuccino proud and, by the way the muscles in her throat were contracting, I guessed she was working up another mouthful ready, it seemed, to send it our way. All the time she remained couched, her knees resting in the straw with her hind legs played out behind, soles uppermost. I knew camels had two toes on each foot – I hadn't watched *Lawrence of Arabia* three times for nothing.

Kevin was pointing to one of them now. 'I reckon it's her right hind foot. She's been favouring that leg these past couple of days.'

'Can you hold her for us?' asked Crystal, putting down her bag.

'Depends on her mood. Some days she plays up and you can't get near her.' Kevin extracted a head rope from his dungarees. 'But we can have a go.' He began walking up to her, whistling through his teeth. 'Hello, Cleo. You going to be a good girl for us today?'

Her neck arched and she swung round baring a set of broken yellow teeth before a stream of semi-digested cud showered out and splattered down Kevin's front. Clearly this was going to be one of her 'bugger off you lot' days.

'And good morning to you too, you old cow,' said Kevin, wiping his beard.

She lunged out again, this time emitting a deep guttural roar which tailed off in to a bubbling rumble as another lump of cud was prepared for ejection. Kevin nimbly jumped back and whistled. 'Not one of her better days, I'm afraid,' he said.

That was all too obvious. Even though we weren't climbing on that hump of hers, we were in for a bumpy ride. Clearly this Cleopatra was missing her Anthony.

'We could sedate her, I suppose,' mused Crystal. 'But I'd rather not unless we absolutely have to.' She edged towards Cleo's hindquarters. There was a twitch of a tail and a flurry of urine stained straw flicked into the air. Cleo swung round with another determined lunge. 'Nope. We're going to have to restrain her somehow,' muttered Crystal, stepping back.

'I'll call the two lads over and see if they can help us,' said Kevin and put two fingers in his mouth. The piercing whistle that he emitted would have shocked even Liza. It certainly gave Cleo something to chew over. Her jaws suddenly ground to a halt and her bottom lip dropped, strings of saliva hanging from it.

Within minutes the two lads had appeared. For some reason I'd been expecting two strapping young keepers with enough muscle power to help wrestle Cleo into submission. What I saw clambering over the gate were two miniature Kevins, minus the glasses – youngsters of about twelve, of slight build, each with an identical mop of Kevin's shaggy black hair.

'Meet the twins,' he said. 'Ben and Barnaby.' The three of them standing together looked like a set of chimney brushes. 'Right, boys,' continued Kevin. 'Cleo's having a strop.'

'What's new,' piped up one of the lads.

'Anyway, you know what to do. It's worked before. So let's give it a go now.'

The three of them spread out round Cleo's head, sufficiently out-of-range of her teeth though not from the spit that came flying out in all directions like an out-of-control garden sprinkler, and what cascaded through the air was green and lumpy and smelt as evil as an unemptied dog litter bin on a hot day.

But it didn't deter the three of them. They bobbed and weaved in front of Cleo, each clapping and calling for her attention. Ben and Barnaby really got into the swing of things, jumping up and down, like jacks-in-a-box, waving their arms above their mops of curls.

'Cleo ... here!' shouted Ben – or was it Barnaby?

She swung in his direction.

'Cleo ... over here!' shouted Barnaby – or was it Ben?

If Cleo wasn't confused I certainly was.

But the twins were enough of a distraction to enable Kevin to eventually dart forward, grab her head collar and clip on the rope. And with her head once restrained, she immediately calmed down though she still continued to puff out her cheeks and utter low rumbles of anger.

Now it was the turn of us two vets to step in. We did so with caution, both Crystal and I wary of the beast even though Kevin now had her head firmly secured and held close to his chest. There was still the risk of an almighty kick from one of those back legs should Cleo chose to strike a blow for camel's lib.

'Which foot did you say it was?' queried Crystal, bending over, hands on her knees, peering down at the camel's hind legs, half-buried in straw.

'Her right,' said Kevin, scuffling forwards as Cleo tried to pull away. 'Hold still, you bugger,' he added with a whistle.

'OK, Paul, let's see what we've got here.' Crystal crouched down alongside Cleo's massive thighs and reached down to pull the straw away from the camel's upturned toes.

I shuffled up next to her. 'Careful now,' she warned, 'in case she kicks out.' I quickly shuffled back a pace or two. No need to be too heroic here. I was no Lawrence. Though the thought of Crystal and I tumbling into the straw together was not without its attractions.

'Guess there's the reason for her lameness,' said Crystal, her finger circling above the sole between the claws of Cleo's right foot. The area was swollen, the skin red and angry-looking.

'An abscess?' I said, peering over her shoulder.

'I should think so. Probably the result of a puncture wound.'

Kevin chipped in. 'You going to lance it then?'

I looked down at Crystal.

'Yes,' she said. 'That's the idea.'

Kevin gave a long whistle. 'Right, lads,' he said, turning to the twins, 'you both stand out of the way. Like Maggie Thatcher, this lady's not for turning.'

For a moment I thought he was referring to Crystal who indeed did have a very determined look on her face. But he was talking about Cleo. He now had his right arm tucked around the back of her head, his hand holding on to the head collar on that side. Her chin he held close with his left hand, still clutching the head rope, the end of which was wrapped round his wrist. If Cleo was going to lunge, Kevin was going to take the lunge with her.

With the instrument pack unwrapped at a distance judged to be safely out of kicking range, disinfectant was splashed onto the affected sole. Cleo gave a low grumble and shifted her weight – all 500 kilos of it – her brown mountainous hump tilting towards us.

'Just watch out,' warned Crystal.

I'd taken out a scalpel handle and attached a blade ready to give to Crystal but wisely put it back until required. She had now edged back over Cleo's right foot and was about to prod the swollen sole to locate the spot where the skin pitted most – the spot to plunge in the blade.

Despite her warning, despite the fact we were all tensed and ready, we were still unprepared for the ferocity of Cleo's reaction to having her foot prodded, however gently. There was an agonized bellow. Her right leg thrashed out in a cloud of straw. Crystal was knocked back into my arms. Oh what a moment. A moment to be cherished. Crystal enfolded in my arms. The warmth of her body, her delicate perfume so close. The fantasy was fleeting.

'Shit,' she exclaimed and quickly extricated herself from my embrace. Her chest was heaving. So was mine.

Cleo's leg was now sticking out in the straw.

'Hey, Dad, we'll sit on her,' chirruped Ben and Barnaby.

'I'm not sure that's a good idea,' said Crystal who, having brushed herself down, had recovered her composure.

'What the heck,' whistled Kevin. 'They'd enjoy a bit of a rough and tumble.'

They're not the only ones, I thought, as my heart continued to race from its close encounter with Crystal.

'Go on, boys. But be careful,' Kevin added.

The twins darted forward and each of them straddled Cleo's back leg, clinging on as if preparing themselves for a rodeo.

'Oh very well,' said Crystal, sounding far from enthusiastic.

I was keener. After all it could mean another chance to save (make a grab for) Crystal; all in the name of professional duty.

I handed her the scalpel and backed away. But not too far. I didn't want to miss her if I did need to make a grab for (save) her.

'Here goes then,' she said glancing round. 'Hold onto your horses.'

Camels, Crystal, camels.

She palpated the sole once again. Cleo roared. Her thigh muscles trembled and bulged. But the two lads held on grimly, rocking up and down and from side to side.

Then in plunged the tip of the scalpel and out poured a fountain of pus. Cleo shrieked again. She wrenched her head round, trailing Kevin with her. She gave a massive kick. The boys bounced off. Crystal reeled back. My arms opened wide.

Yes, yes, yes, I'm here, Crystal. I'm here.

Ben and Barnaby fell into them.

By the time we had sorted ourselves out, Cleo had staggered to her feet and was standing, her sides heaving in and out like bellows, her head covered in sticky green foam. But Kevin was still hanging on, dangling from her head rope.

'Just hold on a mo,' said Crystal. 'We need to give her a shot of antibiotic.' The twins meanwhile had skipped round to the front of the camel none the worse for their tumble, and were ready to distract Cleo again if necessary. But it seems we had knocked the wind out of her sails as she stood there, motionless, while Crystal plunged a massive dose of long-acting penicillin into her thigh.

'One down and one to go, I believe,' said Cleo, slapping Cleo's rump, clearly in her element, clearly enjoying herself.

Our next port of call was a large pen totally enclosed in mesh, fitted out with wooden perches, swings, and tyres suspended from chains. Clearly not kitted out for the likes of guinea pigs or rabbits. And a bit OTT for budgerigars. So for what, I wondered?

Leading off from the pen was a small tunnel, screened by a rubber flap, which gave access to a shed. It was from this shed that came a muffled volley of squeals and grunts.

'Sounds as if Mitchell's up to his old tricks again,' said Crystal, striding over to the side of the shed and giving it a hefty thump.

Hey? What was this? Me? No, of course not. Just that whatever was in the shed just happened to be called Mitchell.

Mmm. Mitch the meerkat? Mitch the mongoose? Mitch the mouse? Oh, no. Surely not Mitch the mouse? I cringed at the thought.

Fingers curled round the bottom of the flap and lifted it a fraction. A pair of yellow-grey eyes peered out.

Crystal thumped the shed wall again. 'Come on out, big boy.'

Ah, this sounded more like it. Mitchell was a big boy then. More of a mighty Mitch.

Crystal rattled the lock on the door. That did the trick. Out shot a lanky-bodied monkey with ginger-brown fur and long, straight tail carried erect.

'That's Melinda,' Kevin informed me.

She was closely followed by two more monkeys, one hugging a baby close to her chest.

'Maureen and Mavis,' I was told. 'Mitch's harem.'

Hmm. This was getting interesting. My namesake was obviously a full-blooded male.

'And here's the beast himself,' said Kevin, as a large, well-muscled monkey with a gleaming gingery coat, padded out through the tunnel. Well, now. What a fine fellow this Mitchell was. Yes. Indeed.

He stood up on his back legs stretching himself to his full height exposing himself; in doing so it was obvious why he was called a big boy. Wow. He put me to shame. He wiggled his eyebrows at us and gave a short staccato grunt before dropping onto all fours again to nonchalantly saunter into the pen.

The female with the baby gave a whimper of fear and made a dash for the tunnel. In a flash, Mitch leapt across and pounced on her back, sinking his teeth into her shoulder. She let out a scream and cowered in submission on the ground, rump in the air.

'Hey! Hey! That's enough of that,' cried Kevin, emitting a shrill whistle and rattling the mesh.

Mitch let go – the female shooting into the shed while he glowered at us. He then sprang. He hit the mesh with a violent crash, gripped it with both hands and shook it, teeth bared in a malevolent grin.

'Ah, you're a right show-off,' declared Kevin, unperturbed.

Mitchell continued to grimace, displaying long, vicious canines, one of which had a broken tip to it.

'That's the problem. See?' Kevin pointed at the blunted tooth. 'And there's that red ulcerated area above it on his cheek. Reckon it's a tooth abscess.'

I was very impressed. He'd reached the same diagnosis as me.

Crystal agreed. 'Means that tooth will have to come out though,' she said, glancing at her watch. 'Look, we're running out of time here. How about Paul coming over later in the week to extract the tooth?'

She looked first at Kevin who nodded his agreement; then at me who was too dumbstruck to move. Me? Crystal was asking me? Wow.

'That's if you want to, Paul,' she added.

I managed to nod. Of course I would. Zoo work? It was something I'd have given my eye teeth for, but now I didn't have to as it was Mitch who would be giving me his.

The following Thursday, I was witness to Kevin's amazing expertise at handling animals. I stood by the trap door of Mitch's pen ready to bolt the flap closed once the females had been run in. This they did as soon as they caught sight of the catching net that Kevin was carrying.

Mitch, in true macho manner, had no intention of being intimidated by the net and even when Kevin entered the pen, he continued to pace up and down one of the perches, raising and lowering his head while emitting a series of threatening grunts.

Spellbound, I watched as Kevin advanced, waving the pole of the net in front of him. Mitch backed along the perch and then swung onto the mesh, still grunting, clearly annoyed. I saw Mitch sink back on his legs, ready to launch himself over Kevin's shoulder. But his move had been anticipated and as he took that flying leap, Kevin whipped the net over the monkey's head, swiping sideways so that the net crashed to the floor of the pen, Mitch hopelessly entangled inside it. Putting one foot on the pole to anchor it, Kevin pulled the net down tight so that Mitch was pinned to the ground.

'Right. He's all yours now,' he declared, with a grin and a whistle.

It was easy enough to jab the anaesthetic through the netting and within minutes Mitch had succumbed; and untangled from the net, we soon had him stretched out on a table in a nearby feed room.

'Bloody big,' commented Kevin. I thought he was referring to Mitch's canines, the broken one of which I was fingering, thinking it could pack a punch if rammed into one of his females. But Kevin had been looking at Mitch's nether regions to which the same attributes could have applied.

I unrolled the pack of dental instruments, and once I'd eased a scalpel blade up round the gum margins of the broken canine, used a dental elevator to prise up the sides, twisting it up and down, gradually loosening the tooth. There was a sudden crack as its root parted from the jawbone. I reached for the dental extractor, gripped the tooth and wiggled it back and forth. Then yanked. Out came the tooth with a satisfying plop leaving a well of blood into which I quickly rammed some cotton wool.

'What do you reckon?' I was eyeing the other canine. The tooth. The whole tooth. And nothing but the tooth. It seemed a pity to remove a sound one. But on the other hand it meant that there would be less severe bite wounds to deal with whenever he attacked the females. Which I understood was quite often – his way of showing who was boss.

'If in doubt have it out,' said Kevin simply.

The second canine wasn't so easy to extract being well cemented in its socket. But after many minutes of sweating, ever fearful the chisel might slip and shoot up through Mitch's mandible, cracking the bone, I managed to pull it off – or rather out – and waved the tooth with its long root at Kevin, proud of my achievement.

'Why don't you keep it as a souvenir,' he suggested.

What a good idea. Have it mounted in a silver clasp to hang round my neck? No fangs. Too fanciful. Too chav-like. But keep it, yes.

As I'd now cut my teeth on some exotic work, it would be something to remind me of this day. Something to look back on when, in many years to come, I too got long in the tooth.

Chapter 17

One of the questions I'd asked at my interview back in June was 'Is there any large animal work?'

Eric had been rather vague in his reply: 'Not much to speak of.'

In one respect he had been right. There wasn't a great deal to speak of. But what there was you could have spoken volumes about; the Richardsons with their darling Clementine; Jill and Alex Ryman with Miss Piggy and her dozen piglets; not to mention the headline grabbing antics of Gert and Daisy – the saddlebacks belonging to Mildred Millichip. It was enough to cope with. I didn't relish more. Not for me the midnight calving or lambing; arms up backsides of cows trying to determine whether they were pregnant or not; nor the tedium of TB testing. Give me Miss Millichip any day – even if it meant contending with that wretched new veterinary dictionary of hers.

It was Beryl who first mentioned the Stockwells. Madge and Rosie Stockwell. Yorkshire lasses – sisters – who'd moved south some thirty years back. They owned a small farm – Hawkshill – tucked into the sides of the Downs between Ashton and Chawcombe.

'A picturesque place by all accounts,' said Beryl, standing by the back door in a fug of cigarette smoke. 'Bit of a time capsule. Rare to find these days.'

I was told the Stockwells had a motley collection of sheep and twelve Jersey cows – remnants of more prosperous times when they managed a large flock and herd of both.

'Never too sure how Eric came to be involved with them,' Beryl went on. 'Something to do with a ewe he found lying on her back when out walking one afternoon. The Stockwells saw him struggling with her. Never like to probe too much as you never know what you might turn up. Best to turn a blind eye to it all.' That was easy for

Beryl with hers. But God knows what she was bleating on about. I reckoned she'd been reading too many tales from the Australian Outback.

Anyway, it seemed an 'association' – as Beryl put it – between the Stockwells and Eric had been forged that day. And he'd been attending to their needs ever since. Often slipping over there when it was quiet at the practice. She imparted that final piece of information with a look that suggested you couldn't pull the wool over her eyes – or rather her one eye.

Still, shaggy dog stories or not, I wasn't bothered. If it helped to keep me away from their animal work, then all to the good as far as I was concerned. In the first five months at Prospect House, that's how it stayed. I had no involvement with the Stockwells. Until one weekend in late November.

The call was from Lucy who was on telephone duty at the hospital that Saturday afternoon. The mere sound of her voice filled me with dread. Not at what was likely to be said – some road accident or whelping bitch – no – just the fact that it was Lucy.

We'd hit another sticky patch in our relationship, like the one a few months back. Lucy was going through one of her self-doubt periods again, not, I think brought on by any problems in her working relationship with Mandy, that seemed to be fine, but to do with us. Her and me. We'd had a couple of rows sparked off by something petty. Isn't that always the case? Blame it on the pressure of work. We both got stretched at times. Both got snappy. Me so more than her. During our last row I'd told her to clear out if she didn't like it. Move back to Prospect House. I think she would if it hadn't been for the animals. As it was she volunteered to do more and more phone cover which meant staying overnight and weekends in the hospital flat. We were barely speaking except when duty called. Like this very minute.

'There's a cow down at Hawkshill Farm,' she said bluntly.

Come on, Lucy, I thought. You can do better than this. Who are we talking about? As I asked the question, bells began to ring. Wasn't it the Stockwell's farm mentioned by Beryl? Yes. Lucy abruptly confirmed it.

A cow down eh? Not very specific. Could be due to a number of things. Uhm … er. I glanced up at my bookshelf as I put down the phone having scribbled down Lucy's terse directions of how to get there. My file on cattle medicine sat on the shelf unopened since I'd left college. No time now, Paul, for freshening your memory. You'll just have to make do with what you can recollect. Cow down. Hmmm.

I started making a mental list of possibilities as I drove the short distance from Ashton before turning off onto a narrow lane that meandered up the northern slopes of the Downs. 'Second gate on the right. And be sure to close it after you,' I'd been told. I found the gate easy enough. A five-bar bleached wooden one that had seen better days. Its five bars were now four; and it was in danger of becoming a three-bar gate if the looseness of the bar I was now pushing to open it was anything to go by.

The gravel track ahead curved round the slope of the Downs and dipped out of sight. Ahead, tucked below the brow of the hill, I could see the upper third of a roof, the red tiles wet and glistening in the watery afternoon sun. Beyond stretched the weald, a patchwork of fields, hedgerows and woods, punctuated by the spire of Chawcombe church, the rectory just visible in the trees alongside. No doubt Liza was in there entertaining Revd Venables at this very minute. The raucous scream of a passing gull reminded me just how painful that entertainment was likely to be.

Having secured the gate as best I could – it meant slipping a rusty chain over the gatepost as the gate had dropped and couldn't be bolted – I drove down the track.

Hawkshill Farm unfolded before me. Beryl had been right. It was a time capsule. Apart from a couple of telegraph poles crossing the fields up from the main road and the distant hum of traffic on that road to remind you of the twenty-first century, you could have been stepping back 300 years. The front of the farm facing me was flint walled, set between courses of red brick, with small-paned, white-framed windows in brick surrounds either side of a wide panelled oak door, weathered grey. The dark twisted branches of some climber – wisteria? – hung over the door, its drooping tendrils swaying in the breeze. To each side of the door a wide flower border ran the length of the building. Though bare, it looked well tended; shrubs pruned, stalks of dead herbaceous plants cut back, the ground freshly dug and dark with manure. No intrusive modern conservatory was stuck on the side; no TV aerial or satellite dish adorned the two red brick chimney stacks at either end; nothing marred the sense of having slipped back in time.

As I drove into the brick-paved yard at the side I half-expected to find a cart-horse peering from one of the stable doors and a hay wain over in the corner. Instead a Landrover was parked there – albeit an ancient, mud-splattered green one; and next to it a bright yellow Smart car. But no sign of anyone. The only sound was the occasional lowing from the oak tithe barn which linked the stables to the house. All the buildings were clay tiled and though some tiles had slipped and many were covered in lichen, they, combined with the oak beams of the barn and the knapped flint of the stables, created a picture-postcard charm, the rustic qualities of which would have done justice to a Thomas Hardy novel. *Far From the Madding Crowd* perhaps? Any minute, Bathsheba – especially as played by Julie Christie in the film – could have walked out of that barn, striding gracefully across the yard to meet me, her golden hair tumbling round her shoulders.

Instead, a short, dumpy figure shuffled into view as I got out of the car. She had a round face with a tomato soup complexion and mousy brown hair in a pudding basin cut.

'Ah, thought I heard a car,' she said slowly. 'Told Rosie it could be vet.' Another stocky figure, with similar rosy-red cheeks and same-styled hair, sidled up beside her. Like Tweedledum and Tweedledee, they stood identically dressed in baggy brown cords, shiny at the knees, and green, army-style pullovers pricked with straw. They made no attempt to move.

'You were right, Madge,' said the second figure. 'It were vet.' She turned and disappeared back in the barn.

I assumed the cow I'd come to see was in there. So donning wellingtons and grabbing my black bag, I hurried across, my mental list of diagnoses growing longer with each stride. I blamed that list for my lack of concentration as to where I was going. The cow pat, one of many in the yard was avoidable. But I failed to see it. I put my foot squarely in it, slipped and just about managed to regain my balance before slithering to a halt in front of Madge Stockwell.

Her gnome-like face with its hooked nose, remained impassive. 'Doesn't pay to be in a hurry,' she said. 'Now't gained if vet breaks leg.'

Beryl had said this was typical of the Stockwells. I would always be referred to as 'vet', never 'Mr Mitchell'. Just 'vet' – as if plucked reluctantly from the modern world. Though no doubt it was different for Eric. But then he had a way with them – or at least with their sheep – if Beryl was to be believed.

'And you closed gate?' Madge went on.

I nodded.

'Needs to be kept closed. So now't can get out.'

'Yes … yes … now this cow….' I said, trying to inject a bit of urgency into the proceedings. Beryl had also primed me on this aspect of the Stockwells.

'No use hurrying them,' she'd said. 'They live in a world of their own.' 'Quick' it seemed didn't exist in their vocabulary unless referring to the one in your nail bed. Everything had to be done at their pace, thank you very much.

Madge led the way – slowly – to where her sister was standing next to the Jersey.

'She looks in a bad way,' I said, quickly stepping over the cow.

She was lying on her side, legs stretched out, her head back, lolling against the partition between her and the Jersey in the next stall.

'Aye, she's none too good,' said Madge, grinding to a halt, her hands stuffed in her trousers. 'Thought that when I first saw her lying there, didn't I, Rosie?'

'You did, Madge.'

'How long's she been like this?' I asked.

Madge took a deep breath. 'How long would you say, Rosie?'

'Don't know. You found her. What time was that?'

'Don't know. Haven't got a watch on.'

'Oh well, never mind,' I seethed, edging round the incumbent cow. She was unconscious, her long, curling eyelashes firmly locked over her eyes.

'Myrtle's always been a problem cow,' said Madge. 'Haven't I always said so, Rosie?'

'You have, Madge. Always.' Rosie shuffled up to her sister until they were almost shoulder to shoulder.

'Mind you, she's been a good milker,' said Madge reflectively.

'She has that,' said Rosie.

'Very good.'

'Yes very good.'

'And still will be if we can save her. But we need to be quick about it. This is an emergency,' I said, trying to instil some sense of how serious this all was. Here we had a cow that was blowing up before our eyes. Unable to belch and so release the gases building up inside, Myrtle's stomach had started to inflate. Her sides were as taut as a drum, the hair on her hide sticking up in dull, brown tufts. She could die any moment.

'Guess she's blown,' said Madge.

'Guess you're right,' said Rosie.

'Guess she is. Yes she is. YES … SHE …IS.…' I felt like hollering. Calamity Jane had nothing on these two. Whip crack away? You must be joking.

Both sisters continued to look as if the Deadwood Stage had passed them by years ago. Talk about slow coaches.

'You'll have to stick'er,' said Madge. 'Like that sheep. Remember, Rosie?'

'The one that Eric poked?'

'The very one.'

'He did a good job there.'

'He did, Madge. A very good job.'

'He's good with sheep, is Eric.'

'He does have a feel for them.'

'He does. He does.'

'Look ladies,' I intervened, not wishing to hear any more, 'if we don't do something right now we'll lose her.'

'If you're thinking of propping her up it won't work,' said Rosie. 'We've already tried it.'

'We have,' said Madge. 'It didn't work.'

'No it didn't.'

'Stick'er will you?' they both chorused. Both sisters' thick, bushy eyebrows seemed to take on a life of their own as they soared in query.

'Look, I think it best if we try and get some calcium into her first,' I said. From the state of Myrtle's udder – huge, swollen, the teats engorged and sticking out – I'd realized that Myrtle was a heavy milker. This could well be hypoglycaemia – a lack of calcium. In which case.…

'We've got some somewhere, haven't we, Madge?' said Rosie.

'Somewhere. Yes.'

'Where'd do you reckon?'

'Under the sink in the kitchen.'

'Think so, Madge?'

'I do.'

'I'll go and have a look then.'

'No. No. Don't bother. I've got some in the car.' I said in an agitated voice. If I waited for her I could be here until the cows came home – all eleven that would be left if Myrtle snuffed it.

'Hurry … hurry … you youngsters these days always in a hurry,' murmured Rosie.

'Always in a hurry,' echoed Madge, as the two of them watched me shoot out of the barn and return minutes later with a couple of bottles of calcium solution under my arm.

I quickly broke the seal on one and connected the screw cap to a long length of rubber tubing. Clasping the end of the tubing to the side of the bottle to prevent any solution from running out, I stretched out my arm.

'One of you hold this please.'

Neither Stockwell moved.

'You then,' I said to the nearest one, thrusting the bottle at Madge. 'Quick now.'

'Hurry. Hurry. Rush. Rush,' she said, shuffling forward to take the bottle.

Stamping down the sodden straw which Myrtle had churned up when she initially went down, I knelt by her outstretched head. Her neck was stiff and rigid. I'd taken a length of nylon cord out of my bag and now used this to form a noose round her, tightening it so that the jugular vein began to swell – a spongy tube that rolled and pitted beneath my fingers. Checking its position in the groove of Myrtle's neck, pressing and repressing the vein with my fingers, I then pointed a large bore needle towards the cow's head and jabbed it in. A thick jet of blood spurted out, flowed warm and sticky over my fingers, coursed down Myrtle's neck.

'You hit it then,' commented Madge. 'Vet hit it,' she added, over her shoulder to her sister.

'Couldn't miss it. Vein that size,' Rosie replied.

I quickly released the cord and the vein collapsed, the flow of blood dropping to a mere trickle. 'Madge … please.' I clicked my fingers and flicked my wrist.

'Rush … rush,' she muttered, leaning over the cow to hand me the tubing and bottle.

'No … no … just the tubing,' I cried, pushing the bottle back into her hand.

'See? That's what comes of hurrying,' she declared.

'Now hold it up,' I instructed.

'Vet says to hold the bottle up,' said Rosie.

'I heard him, Rosie.' Madge raised her arm with the slowness worthy of a tortoise on crutches.

Once some calcium solution had been allowed to sweep throug the tubing, clearing any air bubbles, I connected the end to th needle and allowed the rest to drain into Myrtle. Throughout, sh remained comatose, unaware of what was going on.

'Calved recently has she?' I nodded at Myrtle's huge udder.

'Three days back, wasn't it?' said Madge, looking at her sister.

'Wednesday,' replied Rosie.

'Well it's Saturday now.'

'Yes.'

'Well, three days then.'

'That's what you said, Madge.'

'I did.' Madge turned to me. 'It was three days ago. Wednesday.

I felt like asking 'Are you sure now?' but this was no time fo irony. Whatever, I think I'd sussed the problem with Myrtle. Havin produced a lot of milk in the last three days – since Wednesday to b precise – it had drained her calcium reserves and brought on th nervous symptoms and the dramatic collapse. This intravenou calcium I was giving should produce an equally dramatic reversal c those symptoms. If I had got it right then Myrtle would be up on he feet in no time.

Myrtle's front legs began to twitch. The lids on the one eye w could see slowly drew back with a flicker of the lashes, though th eyeball remained rolled down, only the white showing. It brough back memories of Beryl's eye after she'd discovered the anaconda i the fridge. What a sight – or lack of it – that had been. When th bottle of calcium solution had emptied, I whipped out the needle.

'Right, ladies, let's give Myrtle a hand.' I grasped the Jersey's fro legs, which, now unstiffened, could be bent under her. 'Tuck her bac legs in,' I instructed. 'Quick. Quick.'

'Hurry … hurry,' muttered the Stockwells, as they eased them selves slowly round Myrtle's rump and with much huffing an puffing folded the cow's back legs under her abdomen.

'Good. Now let's try rolling her into a sitting position.' Th proved easy to do now Myrtle had her legs in their natural positio She still remained bloated, especially her left flank which stuck ou like a large brown bubble about to burst. Rosie saw me looking.

'Stick'er now, will you?' she queried.

'I'm in no hurry to,' I replied.

'That makes a change then,' chortled Madge, digging her sister i the ribs.

But it was true. I wasn't in any hurry. Myrtle needed time to get rid of the build-up of stomach gases herself if at all possible. She shuffled her feet more firmly under her as a deep rumble echoed from the depths of her belly, vibrated up her neck and erupted in a loud belch. I never thought I'd be so delighted at hearing such a sound – even if it did come with the stench of fermented grass which had the three of us back away, hands to our faces. Two more belches with their attendant marsh gas smell wafted from her.

'Looks as if vet won't have to stick'er after all,' said Rosie, the muffled words behind the hand still covering her face tinged with disappointment.

As 'vet' I explained that Myrtle needed more calcium solution under the skin to ensure complete recovery, and proceeded to drain in the contents of the second bottle. Myrtle's head was now raised, swaying from side to side, and her eyeballs had rotated back to normal and were beginning to focus.

'She should be up in an hour or so with no ill effects,' I said.

'There's no hurry,' said Madge.

'None at all,' said her sister. 'Is there, Madge?' she added turning to her.

'That's what I said, Rosie. None at all.'

'No, that's what I said.'

'"None at all" you said.'

'Exactly. So there's no hurry.'

'None at all.'

I left them to it. My task had been completed – after all said and done. Whatever was said, I'd said so. Blimey. This was catching.

Back in the twenty-first century I soon forgot about the Stockwells, caught up in the hustle and bustle of daily life. Even if it was a life without Lucy. She continued to keep her distance, spending more and more time at Prospect House, never keen to discuss our faltering relationship. 'I need space' was her only comment when I tried broaching the subject.

It was a Sunday night – that Ovaltine-smooth time when half-read newspapers blend with comforting period dramas on the box to ensure the evening goes with a soothing rustle. Outside it was a wild, blowy night, torrential rain. Not a night to be called out. Though on duty, I'd earlier tempted fate by treating myself to a take-away curry from a new Indian restaurant that had just opened in Ashton; and with the curry eaten, I was about to curl up in front of the fire I'd lit, ready to watch TV, when the phone rang. I pushed Nelson off my lap – he for the moment being my Lucy-substitute in the cuddle stakes – and with a sigh lifted the receiver. It was Lucy at the hospital.

'I've just had a call from the police,' she said.

Curry or no curry, a hot flush coursed through me.

'A DC Jefferies from Chawcombe. He needs to speak to a vet. Here's his number.'

Before I could say anything she'd rattled off the number and put the phone down on me. Blazing birianis. What had I done to deserve this?

The constable was most apologetic.

'Thanks for calling back,' he said. 'But we've got a bit of a problem with a cow stuck in a gravel pit.' My guts contracted in hot spasms as he went on to explain. Thank God I hadn't chosen the vindaloo.

'Couldn't you get the owners to help?' I asked, desperate to find some way of wriggling out of what sounded like a nightmarish situation.

'They're there now, sir. The Miss Stockwells. They haven't said much. Just that someone must have left their gate open. That's how the cow got out. Told us to call vet. They mentioned your name actually. The young one who's always in a hurry.'

Hmm. Seems I'd been put in the hot seat. Talking of which, the curry.... 'Excuse me, but I must go,' I said hurriedly. 'But I'll be with you as soon as I can.'

DC Jefferies sounded relieved. So was I by the time I left Willow Wren and found my way to the gravel works in question.

I knew the spot. It was across the main road opposite the turning up to Hawkshill Farm. A series of disused gravel pits, some of which were due to be turned into lakes for anglers and trout farming i' granted planning permission. But it was another matter finding the place in the dark with the rain bucketing down, the windscreen wipers barely able to cope, the road awash with water. If it continued at this rate it would be me not the car doing a crawl – swimming fo' safety.

As it was, I nearly missed the turning down to the pits, but th' swirl of yellow water running through a gap in the hedgerow gave clue to its whereabouts. As I plunged in I did wonder whether I wa' being foolhardy. But the DC hadn't warned me of there being an' problem so I ploughed on down the track, skidding through pools o'

chre mud, the engine whining, the car lurching one way then the
ther as the tyres lost their grip and the steering wheel spun in my
ands. I couldn't believe it. Yet again I was finding myself in the hot
eat. And boy was it burning. I clenched every orifice as I careered on
own.

Gradually the sheet of rain ahead took on a fluorescent hue
ondensing into blurred columns of light that became brighter and
righter, sharpening as I drew nearer until they defined themselves
s two banks of floodlights casting an arena of white into which I
plashed to a halt. I found I had joined a fire engine, two police cars
nd a Landrover. Yellow-helmeted figures, their elongated shadows
ndulating across the boggy ruts and banks of sand like black
rooked fingers, were busy unrolling lengths of canvas. At the
erimeter of the corona of lights stood two diminutive hooded
gures, their bodies lost within the folds of identical brown rubber
apes that ballooned from their necks to the ground like a couple of
ells. I didn't need to be told who they were: Madge and Rosie
tockwell.

A man in a dark blue windcheater and peaked cap battled his way
ver to me, clutching his hat. He was drenched through, his trousers
at against his legs. I wound the window down a fraction, delaying
he moment when I had to get out and get drenched too.

'Mr Mitchell?' he enquired, leaning down to the gap.

I nodded.

'DC Jefferies. Grim night to call you out,' he continued, through
lenched teeth. 'But they insisted.' He raised a sodden arm and
ointed in the direction of the two rubber bells.

Another figure, yellow helmeted, dressed in bulky dark-blue
cket and trousers with fluorescent strips down the sides and around
uffs and hems, slipped alongside.

'This is Frankie Woods, Chief Fire Officer,' said the DC.

'And responsible for getting this bloody animal out,' yelled the
fficer, the wind whipping the words away. 'She's being a right cow.'

I don't think he realized a pun had just been made and I didn't
hink it appropriate to point it out. Under the circumstances it would
ave been the pits – with me ending up in one of them.

And that seemed a distinct possibility as the wind buffeted me
bout, knocking me against the car, as I attempted to don water-
roofs and wellies before I was pitched into the full force of the wind
nd rain and dragged across to the edge of a gravel pit.

Only the restraining hand of Frankie Woods stopped me fror
sailing over the bank into the thick yellow morass spread out befor
me, the surface bubbling from the rain beating down on it, the flood
lights picking out the head of the Jersey cow stuck in the middle, th
brown of her eyes a stark contrast to the custard-like slurry cakin
her head. Those eyes were full of fear as she fought to prevent herse
sinking from sight into that cauldron of mud. I could feel my hea
sinking with her. Hell. What on earth was I supposed to do?

Nothing it seemed, as Frankie had everything under control.

Even I was under the officer's thumb – quite literally – as the win
suddenly whipped behind my knees knocking me off-balance; I wa
rescued from toppling into the gravel pit again by Frankie's manl
arm thrown round my waist, pulling me close. It was enough to sta
tongues wagging.

'Just watch it, sir. We don't want to have to pull you out as well
the officer said, gently releasing me.

So I did just that – watch it.

I saw several firemen appear through the rain carrying shove
with which they proceeded to dig away the bank, dollops of yellov
mud flying through the air, making a shallow – if slippery – gull
down to the water's edge.

I began to wonder what use I was here. Well, maybe the cov
would need looking at if they ever got her out. Perhaps that's wh
the Stockwells had in mind when they asked for me. Who knows
They hadn't made themselves known since I'd arrived. What dum
bells.

It didn't take long before the gully had been dug out.

Two firemen stumbled forward, clutching the ends of two canva
strops – as I heard one of the crew call them. One man was als
holding what looked like a long, thin metal ruler with a hook on th
end of it. They waded in, gradually sinking until, waist deep, the
were level with the cow, one each side. Waves of mud lapped alon
the edge of the pit as the man with the metal probe struggled to fee
it under the cow's belly.

'Got it,' cried the other fireman who had been groping for it in th
mud. He drew the probe up, attached the strop to the hook and tol
his mate to start pulling it back under the cow. Once done, th
process was repeated with the other strop; firemen up on the ban
then secured the metal loops on the ends of the strops to a pulle
which had been erected on an anchor post hammered into th

ground. While the two firemen stayed with the cow, the rest of the crew, under Frankie's guidance, got in position to winch the strops up. It was a bit like preparing for a tug-of-war.

'OK lads,' shouted Frankie, above the howl of the wind. 'Shoulders to it. Quick as you can. Hurry up.'

I saw one bell slowly turn to the other and whisper in her hood. One didn't have to be quick off the mark to guess what she was saying.

Within seconds, the slack on the canvas ropes had been taken up. Within minutes, the cow had started to move from the centre of the gravel pit, shouts of encouragement coming from the two men with her. There was a loud glug as her body broke the surface of the mud as first a yellow neck, a shoulder and then a back appeared. All of a sudden, she was lying on the bank like a stranded yellow whale, her flanks heaving, her nostrils spurting clouds of steamy breath.

A cheer went up from the firemen.

'Well done, lads,' cried Frankie, turning to me to give me a hug, holding me a fraction longer than I thought necessary. Excuse me. But what was it with this guy? Were the studs in my ears giving out the wrong signals? 'All yours now.'

'What?'

'The cow … she's all yours.'

She is? I thought. Really? All mine. Standing there, watching the rescue had blotted out any thoughts as to what I was doing here – why I had been called in. It was as if the torrential rain had seeped into me, waterlogged my brain. I couldn't think straight. Certainly I couldn't stand straight as another gust of wind threatened to whirl me away had it not been for Frankie manhandling me again. Oh dear. I was beginning to feel swept off my feet. And I wasn't that way inclined, was I? It was enough to get the wind up me in more ways than one.

It was the bells who brought me to my senses. They'd finally made a move and had edged down to the recumbent cow. I slithered across to my car, collected my black bag and squelched back over to join them.

'Think it's Dilly,' said one.

'Could be,' said the other.

'Reckon so,' said the first.

'Think you're right,' said the second.

Ding dong went the bells together. 'We think it's Dilly,' I was told.

I heard the swish of uniform, the splash of big leather boots confidently stepping down the bank; and then the broad shoulders of the chief fire officer hove into view through the mist of rain, generous lips open, dark eyes full of concern. I felt my legs go weak at the knees as another gust of wind hit them. Could I really be falling for a fireman?

'I've been so concerned for you,' said Frankie, reaching out.

'Well....' I faltered.

'So concerned,' the officer went on, walked straight past me to put one hand on each of the Stockwells' shoulders. 'Not the sort of night for us ladies to be out in.'

A rubbery squirmy noise was emitted by both bells.

Us ladies? It suddenly twigged. What an idiot I'd been. Frankie was a woman fire officer. Thank God for that, as I'd been getting worried. Now perhaps I could stop fretting about my sexuality and concentrate on the job in hand.

I prodded the cow as she lay in front of me like a soggy yellow blancmange. Could she get up? Maybe she had a broken pelvis, a fractured femur, ligament damage.

'Had cow down once,' said a Miss Stockwell. 'Remember, Madge?'

Her sister's cape squeaked. 'I do, Rosie.'

'Vet gave her an injection.'

'Didn't work though.'

'You're right, Madge, it didn't.'

'Didn't work,' said the bell, swivelling to me.

'No it didn't,' the other chimed in.

'Well, maybe this time,' I said, drawing up an anti-inflammatory injection. As I plunged it into the cow's thigh, she gave an almighty bellow, threw herself forward, scrabbled in the mud and thrusting her rump up, kicked out her forelegs and lurched to her feet.

'Well, I'll be damned. That soon worked,' said Frankie with a throaty chuckle. 'Good for you.' I was given another hearty hug which this time I didn't mind a bit.

The problem now was to get Dilly back to the farm. The main road had to be crossed. Though relatively quiet at this time of night and with such foul weather, there was still the danger of being mown down – making mincemeat of Dilly.

But Frankie had thought of that. The main road was sealed off by the police car, fire engine and attendant Landrover, their blue lights lashing to light the way as Dilly was led across, a bell-caped tockwell swishing each side of her. I watched the gate, temporarily epaired to five bars, being pushed open and the Jersey herded hrough. The gate closed and the Stockwells were swallowed up by he night.

'Funny pair,' commented Frankie. 'Seem to live in a world of their wn.'

I nodded, thinking of the time warp sensation I felt when I last alled on them. Which side of the fence was it best to live on? I really lid wonder as engines revved up, lights flashed, tyres screeched away nd when I turned on the radio I was greeted with news of the latest omb alert.

But on this side of the gate were the Cuddles, Clementines and Miss Piggys of the world needing care and attention. And I needed hem just as much as they needed me. They were the drug which cept me addicted to veterinary work. They were my fix.

My only regret at present was that I didn't have Lucy to share that atisfaction with me. Our relationship was floundering in an emotional pit – much like the one the Jersey had been stuck in. A pit hat was dragging us under.

Come on, Paul, I thought, there has to be a way of pulling us out of this mess – strops or no strops.

Chapter 18

We were now approaching the season of goodwill, the time for festive cheer. Christmas. Though the look on Beryl's face as I dragged a Christmas tree into reception could have slayed a reindeer at fifty paces and stopped any bells jingling in their tracks.

'We don't want that thing in here, thank you very much,' she said, casting a jaundiced eye – as we know, her one and only – at the tree I was now propping up against the wall.

'Why ever not, Beryl?' I declared, still full of conviviality, but I could feel my good mood beginning to wither under her gaze. What she needed was a good dose of volts to get her switched on. Lighten her up.

Her glass eye continued to flicker on and off me as she replied. 'The needles make a mess everywhere. And a dog's bound to cock his leg against it. I'm sure Crystal wouldn't approve.'

'What's this? What's this? Did I hear my name being mentioned?' Crystal had swung into reception, bright, bubbly, full of cheer. This was more like it.

Beryl wobbled on her perch. 'I was just saying about the tree....'

'Ah, yes, what a good idea. Just the thing to give the place a bit of festive cheer, don't you think?' Crystal flashed Beryl a smile.

'Well, if you say so....' faltered Beryl.

I picked up the tree and took it through to the waiting-room humming 'We wish you a merry Christmas', conscious of the filthy look Beryl was giving me.

That lunchtime Mandy and Lucy went into Westcott's 'Everything a Pound' store and returned with boxes of lurid purple and emerald-green glass balls and red amorphous plastic figures which could have been angels, elves or Victorian carol singers depending on how they caught the light and at which angle you viewed them.

They set to work festooning the tree with this clutter of tat but found they had underestimated its size and were forced to supplement the decorations with blobs of cotton wool and lengths of white bandage draped across the branches. As a result the tree ended up looking like something Florence Nightingale might have practised on prior to going out to the Crimea – the splashes of red ornaments adding a certain bloody realism.

'No, I think that's going a bit too far,' I said, throwing up my hands when they showed me some blown up latex surgical gloves sprayed with gentian-violet, the idea being to tie them in pairs over the doorways.

However, the tree, despite its wounded appearance, did lend a touch of festive cheer to the hospital. And I certainly needed it to help boost my spirits. For two reasons.

For a start I was going to be on duty over the two days of Christmas. I'd thought it likely being the new boy. So no real surprise. Though to be told in July, only two weeks after starting at Prospect House, did seem a little over eager on the part of Crystal and Eric. Still, there we go.

Then there was the problem with Lucy. A week before Christmas I learnt that she was going to be the duty nurse for those two days. Oh dear. I could foresee difficulties there. Communications between the two of us were still patchy to say the least. We weren't really speaking. Not in the heart-to-heart sense. Everything very much on a neutral footing, Everything on hold. So, wow. What a Christmas I had to look forward to. More woe ... woe ... woe ...than ho ... ho ... ho ... seemed likely.

Crystal called me into the office to discuss the matter.

'I hope you don't think I'm prying, but how are things between you and Lucy?' she asked.

I outlined the situation without going into too many details. I had been warned not to let it interfere with work. But then I didn't think it had. Both Lucy and I had got on with what was needed to be done each day without the atmosphere becoming too strained. Though obviously there'd been enough tension for Crystal to have picked up on it. Probably Mandy had kept her informed. Sweet girl.

'Thing is, Paul,' Crystal went on, 'the Christmas duty roster means the two of you will be working on your own together. Do you foresee that being a problem?'

'Don't see why it should be. We've managed so far.'

Crystal tapped her nails on the desk. Those neat pink shells. So dainty. She continued to tap. Clearly something was on her mind. 'Eric and I have been discussing the phone cover. In past years we've always had the calls diverted to our home number and assume you'd like to do the same and have them put through to Willow Wren this Christmas.'

I shrugged. 'Fine by me.' As I said it I suddenly realized what she was getting at. Of course. What would Lucy do? By having the calls diverted there was no excuse for her having to stay at the hospital those three nights like she had been doing these past few weeks whenever she was on duty. She could just as easily be with me at Willow Wren, only needing to go in to see to the few remaining in-patients each day and to help me out with any emergencies should they arise.

'I'll leave it to you to work out the best arrangement,' concluded Crystal tactfully.

With three days to go before Christmas Eve, Lucy still didn't give any indication of what she was going to do.

'Haven't decided,' she said, when I tackled her about it. 'Anyway, what's it to you whether I stay at the hospital or not?'

She stormed away before I had the chance to say that it actually mattered a great deal. I couldn't imagine me spending Christmas alone at Willow Wren and her in a similar situation at Prospect House. Especially now she didn't have to. It seemed absolute madness. And yet it looked as if it was heading that way.

With two days to go before 'crunch time' there was the hospital's Christmas party to get through.

Not being on duty that evening, Lucy had come back to the cottage when evening surgery finished. I almost wished she hadn't bothered as her mood was so foul.

We both got ready for the party in stony silence. She wore black trousers and a turquoise halter neck blouse, her fair hair done up in a chignon, and to me looked absolutely stunning. I did try to compliment her but merely got a curt 'Thanks' in reply. So be it, I thought, as we drove over the Downs to the hospital.

It seemed the party was always held at Prospect House. I had had visions of a slap-up meal at one of the many fine restaurants of which this part of West Sussex boasted.

'No, no,' Beryl had told me. 'That wouldn't be appropriate. Some of the practice's long-standing clients get invited, you see.'

'What, for drinks round the operating table?' I said.

'Goodness, no way,' said Beryl, not realizing I'd been joking. I imagined it would be off-putting for a client to have nibbles where Tibbles had been castrated. It was drinks in the waiting-room instead, the bandaged tree a focus for the small-talk.

'I think it's cleverly done,' enthused a man in velvet jeans, with bleached spiked hair and a silver cross tangling from his right earlobe. 'Very, very, allergoric. I can see how it alludes to pain and suffering. The healing of wounds. The spread of care through the branches of life. Splendid. Very well thought out.'

Not wishing to be lumbered with the likes of him, I quietly moved away.

'Hello, Mr Mitchell.' I turned to find George and Hilary Richardson standing behind me.

'So how's Clementine?' I asked, after pleasantries had been exchanged.

'Oh she's in fine fettle,' said George Richardson, smoothing down each end of his moustache in turn. 'And the foal's an absolute poppet.'

'Actually, we've a little something here to remind you of that evening,' said Hilary, handing me the gift-wrapped parcel she'd been holding. 'A "thank you" from Clementine.'

When I opened it later, I found I'd been given one of the mare's old shoes, polished, with 'Love from Clementine' painted in gold round the edge. Yes … well.

'Consider yourself lucky,' Beryl said. 'The Richardsons don't usually part with anything belonging to her.'

The Rymans too bore gifts. A pound of sausages for each of us – pork, of course. 'Miss Piggy's half-sister,' Alex informed us cheerily. Beryl promptly dumped hers on me.

With the arrival of Miss Millichip, the Rymans and her had a topic of common interest; and like pigs round a trough they tucked into the canapés with snorts and snuffles of enthusiasm as the merits of porcine husbandry were chewed over.

Beryl had invited Cynthia Paget who shunted me into a corner of reception and repeatedly poked me with a cocktail stick as she enumerated on the virtues of her new young lodger, down for the pantomime season, starring in Westcott's production of *Aladdin*, alongside Francesca Cavendish.

'He's been on TV, you know,' Mrs Paget informed me. 'Played a corpse in an episode of *Midsomer Murders*, so he tells me. Against stiff opposition for the part too. Such a sweetie. I've allocated all of my freezer space to him. Can you imagine?'

Obviously the chap had been rubbing Mrs Paget up the right way. Only hope she didn't eventually get on his wick.

Revd Venables and his wife also made a brief appearance on their way through to a carol service in the Festival Hall.

'How's Liza doing these days?' I enquired above the hubbub of voices.

'Sorry, didn't quite catch that,' said the reverend, cupping a hand round his left ear.

'He's getting a bit hard of hearing,' confessed his wife. 'I blame it on all the ear plugs he keeps shoving in his ears. Bound to cause some blockage.'

'What's that, dear?'

'Mr Mitchell's asking how Liza is.'

There was a shake of his head.

'Liza,' I said louder, leaning closer to him. 'The cockatoo.'

The vicar flinched visibly. He drew back and, with a trembling hand, snatched up a cheese and pineapple cocktail and popped it quickly in his mouth, snapping the stick between his fingers. His wife answered for him.

'Oh she's fine, Mr Mitchell. Always in such good voice. Charles wouldn't part with her for the world,' she said, turning to him. 'Would you, dear?' she bellowed in his ear.

The reverend's head shook even more violently and he seemed to cross himself. Or maybe he was just scratching his chest.

Eric bounced between clients, sloshing wine into glasses, thrusting peanuts at people, his bald head glowing, his red nose a challenge to any reindeer, Rudolf or otherwise.

Crystal looked divine in a soft suit of muted grey with a filigree of gold around her neck matching the delicate earrings that hung from those wonderful petite earlobes of hers. She glided demurely through the gathering, a nod here, a word there, a longer conversation with the Richardsons who handed her a horseshoe-shaped present which she accepted with gracious ease. A queen among her courtiers. A Guinevere. Me, one of her knights in shiny armour. Clang.

I caught Lucy's eye and was jousted out of my reverie: the look she threw me enough to unseat the hardiest of knights. It reminded me of the problem we were still saddled with; and it quickly brought me down to earth with a bump. Felled. Rather like what happened to the Christmas tree.

During afternoon surgery on Christmas Eve there was an almighty crash from the waiting-room accompanied by the wails of a cat and some frenzied yapping. I rushed through to find the tree had been toppled by a frightened cat trying to scale it and several dogs were scuttling through the pile of needles while a boxer was cocking his leg against the upturned trunk.

'Told you it was a bad idea,' crowed Beryl from her perch in reception. In the mood I was in, that scrawny neck of hers was a sore temptation for being throttled.

With Mandy having already gone off-duty, it was Lucy's restraining hand, dustpan and brush in the other, which calmed me down with a 'Take no notice of her,' softly whispered. Between us we righted the tree, ignoring the panting and slobbering dogs around us.

Once it was straightened and secured in its bucket, we stood back and looked at each other. Maybe that guy with the bleached spiked hair had been right. Maybe the decorations on this tree were allegorical – standing, as he said, for wounds being healed. Our wounds. The emotional wounds between Lucy and me. The look Lucy gave me suggested he'd been talking a load of rubbish. Absolute trash. She was clearly still needled.

By the end of the afternoon's consultations, I was frazzled. So much for heavenly bells ringing out with glad tidings, the practice phone just wouldn't stop ringing with problems of no comfort or joy.

A Mrs Moody brought in a poodle whose top-knot was tied with tinsel and red ribbon.

'Lulu's sliced her paw on a broken decoration,' she said, full of Christmas spirit, and gave a little burp to prove the point.

There followed a Jack Russell who had seized the chance to wolf down half-a-dozen chocolate angels and whose innards were now pinging like discordant heavenly harps.

The last patient was a Persian brought in a cat basket festooned with gold ribbons and a tiny Father Christmas tied to the bars. She'd been caught gnawing at a defrosting turkey and was now being sick.

I wondered what Father Christmas had in store for me the next day. A lame Rudolph with an infected hoof?

'And you too,' sighed Beryl as the last client wished us yet another

'Happy Christmas' and was ushered out of reception, the door locked rapidly.

'Streuth,' declared Eric, rolling out of the other consulting-room, sweating profusely. 'Let's hope for your sake that's it for now and you have a quiet time over Christmas.' He gave me a rueful look, his eyes flicking to Lucy who had appeared in the doorway. 'The two of you that is.'

'You can call on us any time should you run into difficulties,' said Crystal, striding through from the office where she'd been finalizing some accounts on the computer. 'We'll both be at home.' She too glanced at Lucy. There was an awkward pause.

'Well anyway, happy Christmas everyone,' said Beryl straining forward, presenting her cheek for a peck. We all obliged.

With final best wishes made, Beryl, Eric and Crystal piled out, leaving Lucy and me standing in the empty reception, only the muffled sound of a dog yapping forlornly in the ward to break the silence. And was it going to be just that? A silent night – a night wholly apart?

'Well, Lucy,' I said, hands in my pockets. 'It's your decision. You staying, or coming back with me?' I looked at those hazel eyes, the freckles on the snub nose, the fringe of hair across the brow. Standing in front of me was the best present I could possibly wish for – if only she'd let me wrap her in my arms.

But it seemed my wish wasn't going to be granted. Lucy backed away. 'I think it best if I stay here,' she murmured, averting her eyes.

So be it I thought. But what a crazy, crazy situation.

My mood was still foul on Christmas morning, matched by the frozen chicken I'd forgotten to take out of the freezer when I'd got back to Willow Wren the night before. It was standing stiffly on the draining-board looking as frozen as I felt when the phone rang.

The voice at the end of the line had a thick, Scottish accent and was full of doom and gloom. No Christmas spirit there.

'What seems to be the problem?' I asked, trying to keep the chill out of my own voice once I'd verified that, yes, I was the vet on duty.

'It's Eve ... our British Blue. She's attacked our daughter's moose.'

'What?' I replied, startled by the thought of some moose-savaging moggy stalking round Westcott like Godzilla.

'A moose,' repeated the voice dourly. 'You know, like in Tom and Gerry.'

'Oh, you mean a mouse.'

'Aye, Mickey. Our daughter's pet moose.'

I hadn't much experience in dealing with mice. 'Is he badly injured then?'

'There's only his tail left. She's very upset.'

'I'm sure she is,' I said rather icily, as I pondered over my chicken. 'But you can always get your daughter another one,' I added somewhat tactlessly.

'No … ooo,' drawled the voice. 'It's Eve that's upset. She swallowed Mickey. She's now very poorly.'

'You'd better bring her in then,' I said, jotting down his name before shoving the chicken onto a large plate and placing it on top of the fridge out of reach of Nelson, Queenie and co. who had been circling my legs, looking hopeful.

I rang through to the hospital to warn Lucy that a Mr McBeath would be coming in. Her tone sounded as icy as the bird on the fridge. Talk about being given the cold shoulder.

My mood reflected that of the sick-looking British Blue that turned up on my consulting table half an hour later. She was true to her breed in appearance: dense blue-grey coat, broad-chested, large rounded head with coppery-orange eyes. Though I knew British Blues tended to be calm and collected, Eve was more laid-down than laid-back. She was distinctly off-colour. A miserable moggy that lay on the table without moving, head down, eyes dull, saliva matting the fur round her mouth.

Mr McBeath looked no better. 'We wish you a merry Christmas' had long since died on his lips. Stony-faced and gravelly-voiced, he could have given a block of granite a good run for its money.

'So Eve's being sick?' I asked.

There was a big intake of breath. Mr McBeath exhaled, at the same time emitting a deep, booming fog-horn 'Aye.'

My enquiry as to whether Eve had brought anything up elicited an equally sonorous 'No … ooo'. Mr McBeath was clearly a man of few words.

I gently stood Eve up, where she remained hunched, her short tail dropped. I began to palpate her abdomen, carefully kneading her between my fingers and thumb, pushing my hand towards her spine. A kidney was felt. Her spleen slid past. Loops of bowel. A lump. I

edged my fingers back and felt again. Yes. A lump. I squeezed
cautiously and Eve groaned. I'd found Mickey's mortal remains. Th
fact that Eve was being sick suggested that the mouse was causing
blockage. I explained this to Mr McBeath.

'You do realize we might need to operate.'

'Aye,' he boomed.

'But we'll take an X-ray first if that's OK with you.'

'Aye.'

'So we'll hospitalize Eve now, all right?'

His 'Aye' reverberated in my ears.

'OK, Lucy,' I said. 'Let's see what we've got here.' I'd brought th
cat through to the X-ray room where she'd been laid out, an X-ra
plate under her. We were now ready to take a radiograph of Eve
abdomen.

It all went very smoothly with Lucy working with quiet efficienc
not speaking a word unless spoken to. The radiograph showed
large opaque mass in Eve's intestinal tract.

'See, look, even the mouse's head is visible,' I said, pointing to th
off-white outline of the skull. And Lucy did look, her eyes all at onc
fired with interest.

'Are you going to have to operate?' she asked eventually, turnir
the full force of her hazel eyes on me.

I drew a sharp breath between clenched teeth and said, 'I'm afra
it looks like it. But it won't be easy.' I could see that not only wou
the operation be a tricky one but the cat was in a poor conditio
dehydrated from the constant vomiting so making her a higher ris

Suddenly Lucy's hand was on my wrist. 'It will be fine, Paul. You
see.'

It was too. With autoclaved instruments to hand, a drip set up, th
anaesthetic machine at the ready, Lucy ensured the operation wer
like clockwork. I was impressed with how well she coped. Especial
with no Mandy to oversee her. Our timely intervention ensured th
mouse was removed in minutes; Eve was soon ticking over in th
ward, well on her way to recovery.

'See. What did I tell you?' murmured Lucy.

'But it was only with your help,' I said, turning to her, my han
stretching out, about to brush her cheek when the phone starte
ringing.

'I'll answer it,' said Lucy, backing away, to turn and run out of th
ward.

'You'll never believe this,' she said dashing back. 'A dog's swal-
wed a Christmas stocking.'

She was right. It was difficult to believe. A mouse. Now a stocking.
hat next? A sprig of holly? A cracker or two? Pull the other one,
aul. It was no joke. So, yes, I did found it hard to swallow though it
emed these wretched animals didn't.

'The man on the phone won't listen to any advice from me,' she
ent on. 'Could you have a word?'

Up in reception, I picked up the receiver to be told about the
ocking hung at the bottom of the bed for the wife. She loved
ocolates. Only so did their rottweiler. And he found them first.

'Scoffed the lot,' said the man. 'The stocking as well.'

'Have you tried making him sick?'

'How would I do that?'

'By pushing a lump of washing soda down his throat.'

'I don't think Bismarck would let us near enough to do that.'

I flinched as a growl blasted from the ear-piece.

'Down, Bismarck,' ordered the voice. 'Down. Sorry about that,'
e added. 'He is rather excitable.'

'Well, it might be worth a try,' I urged.

'Uhm. Just a minute then.' There was a brief, muffled discussion
which I heard the word 'vet' before the voice returned. 'My wife
ys she doesn't keep that sort of thing in the house.' There was
other growl and a 'Down, Bismarck'.

'Well, how about some strong salt solution?'

Another growl. 'Down. Sorry?'

'Strong salt solution…?' I faltered, willing to picture the perfect
ene. The man and his wife each side of the passive rottweiler who
ens his heavy, powerful jowls at their command and allows them to
oon the salty solution into the side of his mouth. He licks their
nds gratefully as they finish. Another savage growl thundered
wn the line. 'You'd better bring him in,' I said.

I glanced at my watch. Oh well … bye bye Christmas lunch: hello
e Queen's speech if we were lucky.

Bismarck was a magnificent specimen; gleaming black and tan
at; broad, heavy head; well-muscled body that rippled with
rength.

Mr Dumbrill, in contrast, was a small, spindly chap whose grey
at drooped from his shoulders like the wings on a hunched heron.
he dog was clearly the boss and, taking one look at me, launched

himself across the consulting-room in a frenzy of snarls and slob
bering jaws.

'Hey, where's your Christmas spirit,' I yelled, jumping back t
flatten myself against the wall.

Mr Dumbrill's cries of 'Heel, boy! Heel!' were lost as he an
Bismarck careered round, a jumble of arms, legs and paws, the dog
lead hopelessly entangled between them. Mr Dumbrill twirled an
toppled onto a chair, Bismarck trapped between his knees, bot
owner and dog tied in a cat's cradle of knots.

'Just the job,' declared Lucy, who had just marched in with a larg
lump of washing soda between finger and thumb, a determined loc
in her eye.

She advanced on Bismarck. 'Open!' she commanded, tipping th
dog's head back.

Startled by her fearless approach, his jaw fell open long enoug
for her to flick the crystals over his tongue. There was a firm snap
his teeth as she clamped his jaws shut and vigorously massaged h
throat.

'Swallow, you beast. Swallow!'

Both Mr Dumbrill and I swallowed, and seconds later there wa
an audible gulp from Bismarck.

'I should think so too,' said Lucy.

She had that look in her face – that 'Lucy look' of determinatio
no nonsense. She was in control. No hiding her light under a bush
here. She was positively shining. Glowing with confidence. It put m
in the shade.

Bismarck was now beginning to foam at the mouth.

'Oh dear, are you sure he's not going to have a fit?' cried N
Dumbrill, himself beginning to foam in sympathy, flecks of spitt
appearing at the corners of his mouth.

'No, he'll be fine,' stated Lucy firmly, unravelling the lead ar
steering Bismarck away from the trembling man. 'Now just leave hi
with us so that we can keep an eye on him.'

'Why?' croaked Mr Dumbrill, looking at me.

I was going to say that if Bismarck didn't regurgitate the sock
could block his insides – like that mouse in Eve – and we wou
then have to operate to remove it. But I caught Lucy's look ar
realized it would get Mr Dumbrill into an even bigger flap if I to
him this.

'To make sure he brings the sock up,' I said instead.

While Lucy hauled Bismarck down to the ward, I ushered Mr
Dumbrill out, telling him to stop worrying, go home and tuck into
his turkey. Which reminded me of my frozen bird awaiting me back
: Willow Wren. As I wandered forlornly down to the ward I heard
loud burp. I raced along the corridor.

'Any luck?'

Lucy was backing out of Bismarck's kennel. She stood up, bolted
the door and turned to me. 'Dah ... dah,' she exclaimed
iumphantly, holding up a soggy red stocking.

'Only problem now is where do we hang it,' I joked. The relief
that flooded through me was not so much at the sight of the regur-
itated sock as at the smile that lit up Lucy's face.

When a delighted Mr Dumbrill collected Bismarck later that
ternoon, he handed us a similar red sock – only this one bulged
ith a bottle of champagne.

'For both of you – Merry Christmas!' he cried, as Bismarck
anked the lead and dragged him out of reception.

I held up the bottle. Here was a chance to test Lucy. See how
he really felt. She certainly seemed more relaxed, her mood
appier. Perhaps it was because, with these last two cases, she'd
een able to prove that she really was an efficient, dependable
urse. 'I guess we ought to be celebrating something,' I said,
aving the bottle in the air. My voice trailed off as I studied Lucy's
ce, desperately looking for a clue as to her feelings, some sign of
er new-found confidence. In a whisper, I added, 'A home-coming
erhaps?'

For a brief moment, Lucy's face remained impassive. Then her
es suddenly lit up with renewed sparkle and her lips curved into
at gorgeous smile of hers. 'A home-coming ... yes, that would be
od,' she said and reached up to plant her lips emphatically on
ine.

As we locked up in the dark and crunched down the gravel drive,
m in arm, a rising full moon bathed the front of Prospect House in
wash of luminous grey.

I turned to look at the portico, its pillars like shafts of silver. It had
nly been seven months since I'd first set eyes on that entrance. An
trance that had opened a whole new chapter of my life.

I turned to Lucy.

Moonbeams danced in her hazel eyes.

The look she gave me – that lovely Lucy look – spoke volumes. Of further chapters. More episodes. The prospects ahead looked good. Very good indeed.

As we climbed into the car, I started to hum.

Odl lay ee. Odl lay hee hee.